THE ONLY CHAIR YOGA FOR SENIORS OVER 60 GUIDE YOU NEED:

Chair Yoga for ~~~~~~~ Mobility and
Posture | Bring ~~~~~~~ With Gentle
Sitting Exercis ~~~~~~~ nge Chart |

NOELLE BELL

The Only Chair Yoga for Seniors Over 60 Guide You Need
Copyright © 2024 NOELLE BELL
All rights reserved.

TABLE OF CONTENT

CHAPTER 6:

BONUS # 01:

BONUS # 2:

YOUR FREE BONUS

As an additional BONUS for your purchase, I would like to give you a GIFT.

This is a BALANCED PLATE for breakfast, lunch and dinner!

BALANCED PLATE- the optimal combination of proteins, fats, carbohydrates, vitamins and trace elements in the diet. It is necessary to ensure the normal functioning of the body, and good well-being at the physical and mental level.

HERE you will get not only nutrition recommendations but also

ready-made recipes for a balanced diet that can be immediately used in your everyday life!

Scan the QR code or follow the link

https://amazon-book.minisite.ai/chairyogabonusforseniors

INTRODUCTION

Do you want to reclaim the vitality and independence of your youth? Are you tired of constant aches, pains and limited mobility overshadowing your life? If so then you need a transformative solution that does not involve any grueling workout- the Chair yoga. In this book, your favorite chair will become your gateway to a revitalized life. It is not simply a collection of exercises- but a roadmap to gain your independence, improve your mobility and to get rid of the unwanted pounds, all while sitting comfortably in your chair.

This "Chair Yoga for Seniors" guide is a game changer for you as it will help you unlock a new world of independence. Say hello to newfound self-sufficiency with my tailored chair yoga challenges for beginners and advanced levels. It just takes 10 minutes a day to engage in easy-to-follow yoga poses and exercises that are shared in this book. They will help you regain balance, mobility and vitality effortlessly. Whether you are a beginner or someone who is into yoga, this book offers a whole spectrum of yoga practices that are accessible to all. With just a chair and a willingness to transform, you can start this journey today.

Don't worry! if you don't have any prior experience of yoga. This guide is meticulously created to provide you with clear and step-by-step instructions with illustrations for an enjoyable and rewarding journey. So, don't let your physical limitations define your senior years. Now is the time to embrace a future filled with joy, energy and independence with chair yoga.

CHAPTER 1:
YOGA AND CHAIR YOGA UNVEILED

"Youth is the gift of nature, but age is a work of art."

- Stanislaw Jerzy Lec

With age, we experience reduced flexibility, strength and mobility which makes yoga poses challenging. Chair yoga is the perfect way to address these concerns by offering modifications that can be comfortably performed while using a chair for support. It helps you increase flexibility, strengthen muscles and improve balance, all of which are essential for reducing the risk of falls and injuries. Through chair yoga, you can include mindfulness and deep breathing techniques into your daily routine as well which can alleviate stress, promote relaxation and enhance mental clarity.

EXPLORING TRADITIONAL YOGA PRACTICES

Traditional yoga practices date back to 5000 years and they have evolved over the years. While most people see yoga as just a set of poses it actually consists of a whole spectrum of practices which include physical postures (asanas), breathing techniques (pranayama) and meditation. So, yoga is not just for the body, it is also for the mind. It works its magic by establishing strong mind-body connections and activating neural pathways.

Gentle Exercises (Asanas):

These yoga exercises cover physical gentle movements that help you feel strong, flexible and balanced. These poses are perfect for beginners as they activate the muscles and bones without putting any strain on the soft tissues and ligaments. Some gentle exercises include arm stretches, warrior and mountain pose etc.

Deep Breathing (Pranayama):

Taking deep breaths induces a calming effect on the mind and helps you relax. You can learn simple techniques to take slow, deep breaths that calm the mind, relax the body and give you a boost of energy.

Relaxation:

Living in a super-busy lifestyle, we all need a pause to regain our energies and revitalize. Relaxation practices in yoga help you hit that pause button. It is similar to wrapping yourself in a cozy blanket of peace. It is simply an act of lying down comfortably and letting go of any tension in our bodies. This relaxation allows you to sink into a state of deep rest and relaxation.

Healthy Eating:

Eating well is a way of fueling your body with all the good stuff it needs to thrive. So, choose foods that would make you feel strong and energized, like colorful fruits, crunchy veggies and nourishing grains without relying on any sugary, processed and unhealthy inorganic ingredients.

Mindful Meditation:

Mindfulness is the practice of bringing attention to the present moment. In mindful meditation, the mind is tuned to focus on one single point through paced breathing and visualization.

Meditation is like taking a peaceful stroll through the garden of your mind. You can practice meditation by sitting quietly in a distraction-free environment to find your inner peace and clarity.

BENEFITS OF CHAIR YOGA FOR SENIORS

There are a multitude of chair yoga benefits for people of all ages and abilities. It is highly adaptable and versatile which makes it particularly advantageous for those with limited mobility, injuries or other physical limitations. Some of the proven benefits of chair yoga include:

It improves flexibility: Chair yoga is known for enhancing flexibility due to the gentle stretches in its routine. This can be particularly beneficial for people who experience stiffness due to age or lack of activity. There was this study that was published in the Journal of Gerontological Nursing and it found out that chair yoga significantly improves flexibility in older adults after just 8 weeks of regular practice.

It enhances strength: Despite being seated in a chair, with these poses you can engage various muscle groups in the body. They improve the strength of the muscles, particularly in the core, legs and arms. According to the research published in the Journal of Aging and Physical Activity, chair yoga can increase lower body strength in older adults. The improvement in muscle strength is important for reducing the risk of falls.

It promotes balance and stability: In chair yoga, you can practice poses and exercises that focus on improving balance and stability. This is crucial for people who may be at risk of falls or for those with mobility issues. When the balance poses are carried out in a supported seated position then it can help build confidence and stability. A systematic review published in the Journal of Alternative and Complementary Medicine confirmed that chair yoga can improve balance in older adults.

It reduces stress and anxiety: Like other forms of yoga, chair yoga also adds breathing and mindfulness practices into your routine that can promote relaxation. This is especially beneficial for people who deal with age-related stressors or younger individuals who strive against mobility challenges. A research study published in the International Journal of Yoga Therapy concluded that chair yoga reduces stress levels and improves psychological well-being in adults over 50.

It improves circulation: The movements in the chair yoga exercises are great for stimulating blood flow throughout the body and the better the blood circulation the more improved energy levels and overall well-being you can experience.

It increases range of motion: The stiffness and resistance in mobility that many adults experience after 50 or 60 go away with chair yoga. The gentle movements involved in this program increase the range of motion of the joints and muscles. If you have arthritis or any joint problem then with these light movements you can keep your joints flexible.

It can be practiced anywhere: As long as you have a sturdy and comfy chair, you can practice this form of yoga anywhere. You can do it at home, in the office, or even in a group setting. You don't need to hit the gym or buy expensive equipment to garner the benefits of chair yoga.

It improves cardiovascular health: Since chair yoga is great for blood circulation, it directly improves cardiovascular health. As per the study published in the Journal of Bodywork and Movement Therapies, chair yoga can improve cardiovascular health in older adults by countering high blood pressure and improving heart rate variability.

It enhances cognitive function: Preliminary research also suggests that chair yoga also positively impacts cognitive processes in adults. A pilot study was published in the Journal of the American Geriatrics Society and it found out that chair yoga improves cognitive performance in older adults with mild cognitive impairment.

It offers better sleep quality: Chair yoga is also linked with improved sleep quality in older adults. A study published in the Journal of Alternative and Complementary Medicine confirmed that chair yoga reduces sleep disturbances and improves overall sleep quality in adults with osteoarthritis.

CHAPTER 2:
PREPARING FOR CHAIR YOGA

"You are never too old to set another goal or to dream a new dream."

- C.S. Lewis

Though chair yoga looks harmless and easy to follow, it still requires extra care and caution. When you try different yoga poses and stretches at home, without expert supervision make sure to keep it safe by using suitable equipment. You also need to set up a suitable environment, free from distractions and with enough space to move comfortably. These efforts can only be put in the right direction through a positive mindset which makes you more open and receptive to the benefits of the yoga practice. In this chapter, we will explore various aspects of chair yoga preparation, from selecting the right equipment, creating an inviting practice space and developing the right mindset for a fulfilling journey toward improved well-being and vitality, we will look into it.

EQUIPMENT AND CREATING A COMFORTABLE CHAIR YOGA AREA

A sturdy chair without arms is typically the only necessary equipment for anyone doing chair yoga. However, a quiet, well-lit space with ample room to move freely is also necessary to enhance the overall experience.

Sturdy Chair: First choose a stable and armless chair with a flat seat and a backrest that supports the spine comfortably. Avoid any chair that has wheels or armrests as it may be unstable during yoga practice. On a good chair you can easily sit with your feet flat on the floor and your knees at a 90-degree angle. I would suggest you buy the ones which are most suitable for you. Before making the purchase, try some basic poses on the chair to check if the height and base of the chair are good enough to perform chair yoga with complete safety.

Yoga Mat or Non-Slip Surface: Having a yoga mat or a non-slip surface under your chair is a must to keep it stable during yoga movements. This will help prevent the chair from sliding or shifting during practice for your safety. The mat also gives your feet a nice firm grip while practicing various poses.

Blanket or Towel: Though you don't necessarily need a folded blanket or towel for chair yoga, but there is no harm in keeping them nearby to cushion sensitive areas. You can place them on the chair during certain poses to add extra padding.

Blocks: Sometimes your feet do not reach the ground during certain exercises and you need to keep them on a stable surface, in that case, you can place blocks under your feet to modify poses and provide support. Blocks can be used to elevate the floor for seated poses or to bring the ground closer to you for reaching exercises.

Comfortable Clothing: It is also important to wear loose and comfortable clothing that would allow you to freely move during the stretches. Choose clothing that wicks away moisture to help you stay cool and dry during practice.

LIGHT-WEIGHT RESISTANCE BANDS:

Resistance bands are completely optional, but they can be added to the advanced-level yoga routine to increase the difficulty level and burn more calories. Resistance bands come with varying strengths and you need to choose the ones which are easy and light to stretch. Here are some common types:

- **Thera-bands:** These are elastic bands that are available in various resistance levels, with color codes for easy identification. They are often used for rehabilitation and physical therapy exercises due to their versatility and gentle resistance.

- **Mini Loop Bands:** These are small and circular bands that provide resistance when wrapped around ankles, thighs or arms. They are excellent for targeting specific muscle groups and improving strength, stability and flexibility.

- **Tubing Bands with Handles:** These bands are made of long and flexible tubes with handles on each end. They have adjustable resistance which can be adjusted with the length of the band or by using different color-coded bands. The handles provide a comfortable grip for a wide range of exercises.

- **Figure-8 Bands:** These bands are shaped like the number 8 and they provide resistance when pulled apart. They are particularly useful for upper-body exercises like for chest presses and shoulder raises.

- **Flat Resistance Bands:** Flat bands look like large rubber bands and are known for their versatility. They can be used for resistance training, stretching and improving range of motion.

Quiet and Well-Lit Space: Environment makes a great difference when it comes to yoga. Your mind has to be in a relaxed state and for that, the atmosphere must be calm, quiet and clutter-free. You can create such a place in your home in a room where there are no distractions. Choose a place where there is good light, preferably natural light or soft lighting for a calming ambiance.

DEVELOPING A POSITIVE MINDSET

Your positive mindset is the seed that you plant to reap the benefits of good health. Approach this journey with gratitude, kindness and self-love. You cannot possibly stay fit and healthy if you neglect your nutritional, emotional and mental needs. So, listen to yourself, look into your body cues and then celebrate your efforts instead of focusing on the failures. It is fine if you miss one day of exercise or your health condition does not allow you to practice any certain pose, give yourself the time and space to adjust to the routine. Do not force yourself into anything, be slow, steady and consistent in your efforts and you will see visible results in just 2-3 weeks.

CONSULT YOUR HEALTHCARE EXPERT:

Before starting any new exercise program, it is extremely important to consult with your healthcare provider especially if you have any pre-existing health condition. Pay attention to problems like arrhythmia, osteoporosis, high or low blood pressure, spinal arthritis or bone degeneration and bone spurs as practicing certain yoga poses might be dangerous for people who have those conditions. These conditions require modifications to your exercise routine for the safety of your health.

Let's consider Arrhythmia for instance! In this condition, the patient suffers from irregular heart rhythms which are exacerbated by strenuous exercise. So, in this condition, patients need to avoid activities that suddenly raise their heart rate or cause sudden movements. If you have this condition and would like to practice chair yoga then make sure to get your doctor's approval and discuss your workout routine with him before physically indulging in any exercise.

Osteoporosis is another condition which is common in people over 60. In this condition, bones suffer from weakness and certain exercises may increase the risk of fractures. Though chair yoga can help maintain bone density and strength, it must be done carefully to avoid falls or injuries that could result in fractures. Having a physiotherapist's opinion and recommendation before initiating the yoga program is important. Spinal arthritis or bone degeneration can cause pain and stiffness in the spine, making certain movements uncomfortable or even harmful. Gentle, low-impact exercises that support the spine and improve flexibility without exacerbating pain are recommended for this.

Sudden fluctuations in blood pressure are dangerous for people with hypertension. So, it is essential to keep the blood pressure levels maintained during the yoga exercises and avoid activities that may cause sudden spikes or drops, if you have this condition. If you have bone spurs then consult your doctor first before trying any chair yoga exercise. In this condition, bony growths develop along the edges of bones which cause pain and limit mobility. Your healthcare provider can provide personalized recommendations and guidance based on your health status, helping you to exercise safely and minimize the risk of exacerbating any existing health issues.

CHAPTER 3:
CHAIR YOGA BASICS FOR BEGINNERS

POSES TO WARM-UP

SEATED MARCHING

It is a delightful and effective exercise tailored for seniors to improve lower body strength and promote circulation. This simple yet impactful movement involves sitting in a chair and lifting your knees alternately, mimicking the motion of marching.

Repetitions: 30 seconds

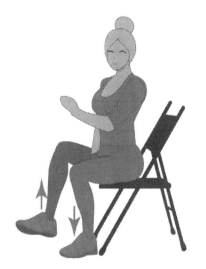 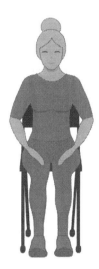 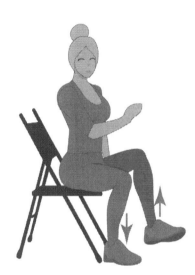

MUSCLES TARGETED

- Hip flexors
- Quadriceps
- Core muscles

INSTRUCTIONS

1. First, sit in your chair in a comfortable position with your back straight and shoulders relaxed.

2. Place your feet flat on the floor, hip-width apart.

3. Lift your right knee toward your chest while keeping your foot on the ground.

4. Lower your right foot back to the floor and repeat the motion with your left knee.

5. Continue this marching motion, lift and lower one knee at a time.

6. Try to match the pace of your movement with the breath while inhaling as you lift and exhaling as your lower

PRECAUTION

Lift your knees gently and avoid sudden or forceful movements.

SEATED ARM REACHES

Seated Arm Reaches provide a simple yet effective way to enhance upper body flexibility and mobility. This exercise is ideal for individuals of all fitness levels and can be performed to alleviate tension in the shoulders and promote a full range of motion.

Repetitions: 3 sets of 12 reaches per side

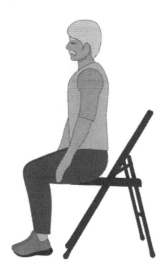 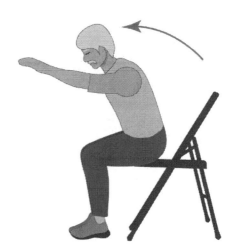

MUSCLES TARGETED

- Shoulders
- Upper back
- Arms

INSTRUCTIONS

1. Comfortably sit in your chair with proper posture and make sure that your back is straight and shoulders are relaxed.

2. Place your feet flat on the floor, hip-width apart.

3. Extend your right arm straight out in front of you at shoulder height.

4. Reach forward with your right hand, stretching your arm as far as comfortable.

5. Hold the reach for a moment, feeling the stretch in your shoulder and upper back.

6. Return your right arm to the starting position.

7. Repeat the motion with your left arm, extending it straight out and reaching forward.

8. Alternate between right and left reaches for a set of 12 per side.

9. Perform three sets, taking short breaks between sets.

PRECAUTION

Carry out the arm reaches with controlled movements to avoid any strain or injury. If you have any shoulder issues, limit the range of motion to a point that is comfortable for you.

SEATED HIGH KNEES

Seated High Knees offer a seated adaptation of the classic high knees exercise, providing an effective way to engage the lower body and elevate the heart rate while remaining seated. This exercise is suitable for individuals looking to improve hip flexibility and strengthen the hip flexors.

Repetitions: 3 sets of 15 lifts on each leg

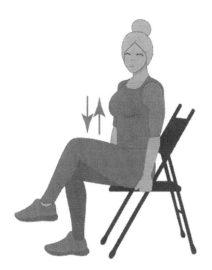 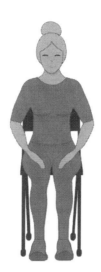 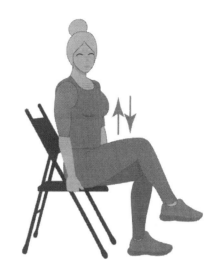

MUSCLES TARGETED

- Hip flexors
- Quadriceps
- Core muscles

INSTRUCTIONS

1. Comfortably sit in your chair with an upright posture and relaxed shoulders.

2. Place your feet flat on the floor, hip-width apart.

3. Engage your core muscles to stabilize your torso.

4. Lift your right knee toward your chest as high as comfortable, keeping your foot off the floor.

5. Hold the lifted position for a moment, feeling the engagement in your hip flexors.

6. Lower your right foot back to the floor and repeat the motion with your left knee.

7. In an alternate movement, switch between right and left high knees for a set of 15 on each leg.

8. Coordinate the high knees with your breath, exhaling as you lift and inhaling as you lower.

9. Perform three sets, taking short breaks between sets.

PRECAUTION

Do the high knees with controlled movements to avoid any strain or injury. If you have any knee or hip issues, limit the range of motion to a point that is comfortable for you. Maintain proper posture throughout the exercise to maximize its effectiveness.

FORWARD FOLD (UTTANASANA)

Seated Forward Fold or Uttanasana, is a calming yoga pose that offers a deep stretch for the muscles in your lower back, hamstrings and spine. This seated variation is accessible for seniors, providing the benefits of a forward fold while sitting comfortably in a chair. The pose is designed to gently release tension, improve flexibility and promote a sense of relaxation.

Repetitions: 2 minutes

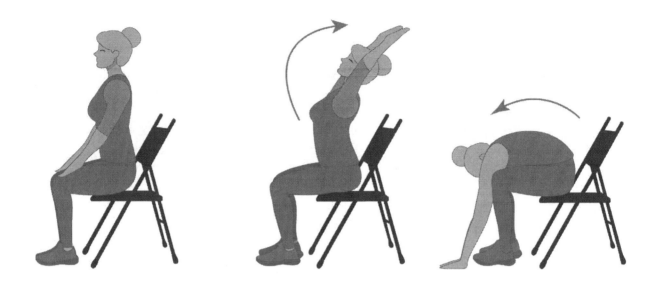

MUSCLES TARGETED

- Hamstrings
- Glutes
- Lower back muscles

INSTRUCTIONS

1. Sit on the edge of a chair with your feet flat on the floor and hip-width apart.
2. Inhale and lengthen your spine, sitting tall.
3. Exhale and slowly hinge at your hips, leaning forward.
4. Reach your hands towards your toes, keeping your back straight.
5. If possible, hold onto your feet or shins; otherwise, use a strap for support.
6. Hold the stretch for 15-30 seconds, feeling a gentle pull along your hamstrings and lower back.
7. Inhale as you slowly return to an upright position.

PRECAUTION

Bend your knees slightly and avoid locking them to protect your lower back.

UPWARD SALUTE POSE

Seated Upward Salute Pose is a delightful yoga stretch tailored for seniors to promote flexibility and enhance overall well-being. This seated variation allows individuals to experience the uplifting benefits of the traditional pose while comfortably seated in a chair.

Repetitions: 1 minute

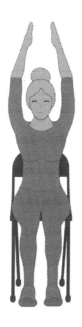
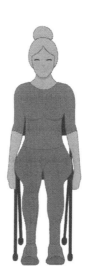

MUSCLES TARGETED

- Deltoids (shoulders)
- Triceps
- Serratus anterior
- Shoulders
- Arms
- Upper back

INSTRUCTIONS

1. Comfortably sit in your chair with your back straight and feet flat on the floor.
2. Slowly take a deep breath and reach your arms overhead with your palms facing each other.
3. Extend your spine as you lift your arms, creating length through your torso.
4. Keep your shoulders relaxed and if comfortable, gaze gently upward.
5. Hold the stretch for 15-30 seconds, feeling a gentle elongation along your spine and through your arms.
6. Exhale as you bring your arms back down to your sides.

PRECAUTION

Rise gradually to avoid dizziness. If you have shoulder issues, keep your arms at a comfortable distance.

SEATED BUTTERFLY STRETCH

This seated stretch is particularly beneficial for seniors looking to improve their range of motion in the lower body and alleviate tightness in the hip area. By mimicking the movement of a butterfly's wings, this stretch provides a comfortable and accessible way to open up the hips while seated in a chair.

Repetitions: 2-3 sets of 5 repetitions

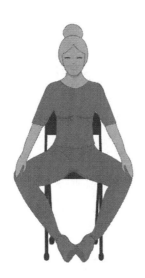 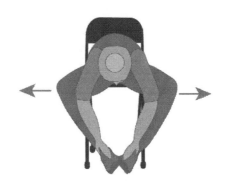

MUSCLES TARGETED

- Adductors
- Inner thighs
- Groin

INSTRUCTIONS

1. First, sit in your chair in a comfortable position with your back straight and feet flat on the floor.

2. Put your hands on your knees and allow your legs to naturally fall outward.

3. Bring the soles of your feet together and allow your knees to drop to the sides.

4. Hold onto your feet with your hands, interlocking your fingers if possible.

5. Inhale slowly as you lengthen your spine, sitting up tall.

6. Exhale as you gently press your knees toward the floor, feeling a stretch in your inner thighs.

7. Hold the stretch for 15-30 seconds, breathing deeply and maintaining a relaxed posture.

8. If you find it challenging to reach your feet, you can put your hands on your knees and use your elbows to gently press your knees down.

9. Release the stretch and shake out your legs to release any tension.

10. Repeat the Seated Butterfly Stretch for 2-3 sets, adjusting the duration based on your comfort level.

PRECAUTION

Take it slow, especially if you have hip or knee concerns. Avoid forcing the knees down; instead, let them naturally descend as you ease into the stretch.

BOW POSE

Seated Bow Pose is a modified version of the traditional yoga pose, adapted for a seated position to provide seniors with a gentle and effective way to stretch and strengthen their back muscles. This exercise is especially beneficial for targeting the muscles along the spine and promoting flexibility in the shoulders and chest.

Repetitions: 5 times

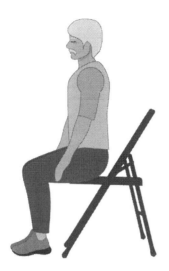 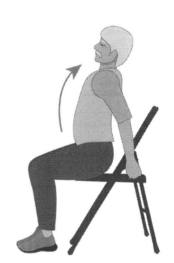

MUSCLES TARGETED

- Back extensors
- Glutes
- Hamstrings
- Back
- Thighs

INSTRUCTIONS

1. Sit in a sturdy chair with your feet flat on the floor and your back straight.
2. Inhale and engage your core muscles.
3. Reach back with both hands and hold onto the sides or back of the chair.
4. Exhale as you gently lift your chest, arching your back while keeping your feet firmly planted.
5. Allow your head to tilt back slightly if comfortable and maintain a comfortable neck position.
6. Hold the stretched position for a few breaths, feeling the opening across your chest and the stretch along your spine.
7. Inhale slowly as you return to an upright seated position.

PRECAUTION

Lift only as much as comfortable and avoid excessive arching of your back and if you have any back issues, modify the pose accordingly.

SEATED SHOULDER OPENER

The Seated Shoulder Opener is a soothing exercise designed to alleviate tension and enhance flexibility in the shoulder area for seniors. This seated stretch can be easily incorporated into your daily routine, providing gentle relief to the muscles around your shoulders.

Repetitions: 5 reps per side

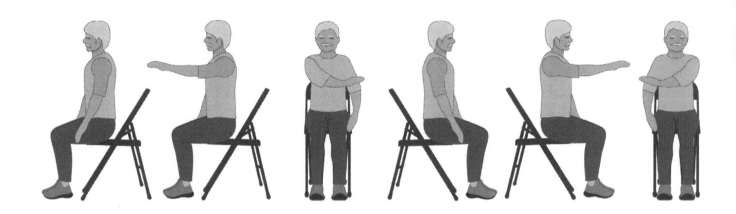

MUSCLES TARGETED

- Deltoids (shoulders)
- Pectorals
- Rhomboids
- Shoulders
- Chest
- Upper back

INSTRUCTIONS

1. Sit in a comfortable chair with your back straight and feet flat on the floor.

2. Inhale and relax your shoulders down, away from your ears.

3. Exhale as you lift your right arm straight in front of you.

4. Inhale and gently reach your right arm across your chest, feeling a stretch in your left shoulder.

5. Hold the stretch for a few breaths, focusing on opening up the shoulder.

6. Exhale as you release your right arm and return it to your side.

7. Repeat the stretch with your left arm, lift it in front of you and reach it across your chest.

8. Hold the stretch, feeling the gentle opening in your right shoulder.

9. In an alternate movement, switch between right and left stretches, moving at a comfortable pace.

PRECAUTION

Open shoulders gradually and avoid pushing beyond your comfortable range and if you have any shoulder issues, modify the stretch accordingly.

SEATED SUNFLOWER STRETCH

Seated Sunflower Stretch is a gentle and invigorating exercise that targets the upper body, particularly the shoulders and chest. This seated stretch promotes flexibility, reduces tension and improves overall posture. It is suitable for individuals of various fitness levels and can be particularly beneficial for those looking to alleviate stiffness in the upper body.

Repetitions: Hold each position for 15-20 seconds, repeat 3 times

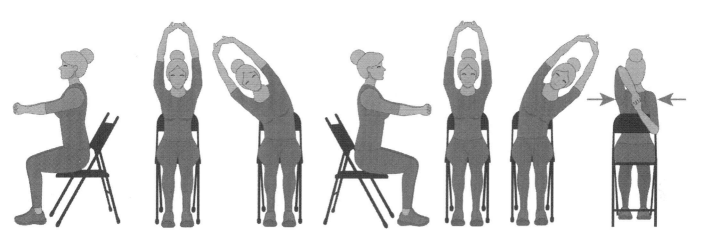

MUSCLES TARGETED

- Shoulders
- Chest
- Upper back

INSTRUCTIONS

1. Comfortably sit in your chair with your back straight and shoulders relaxed.

2. Intertwine your fingers and extend your arms in front of you at chest height.

3. Inhale slowly as you lift your arms overhead, extending them toward the ceiling.

4. Exhale and gently lean to the right, feeling a stretch along your left side.

5. Inhale slowly as you return to the center and then exhale as you lean to the left, stretching the right side.

6. Continue this rhythmic side-to-side motion for a total of 3 sets.

7. After the last repetition, release your hands and clasp them behind your back.

8. Inhale slowly as you lift your chest and arms slightly and squeeze your shoulder blades together.

9. Exhale and relax into the stretch, feeling the opening in your chest.

PRECAUTION

Carry out the stretch with controlled movements to avoid any strain or injury.

If you have any shoulder or back issues, limit the range of motion to a point that is comfortable for you. Maintain proper breathing throughout the exercise to enhance relaxation.

SEATED CROSS PUNCHES

Seated Cross Punches provide an engaging upper body workout, focusing on the arms, shoulders and core muscles. This seated exercise is designed to enhance strength, flexibility and coordination, making it an ideal choice for individuals looking to incorporate dynamic movements into their seated fitness routine.

Repetitions: 15 times per side

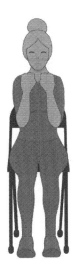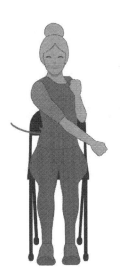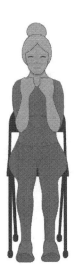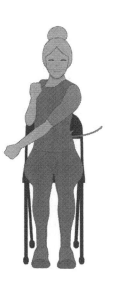

MUSCLES TARGETED

- Arms (Biceps and Triceps)
- Shoulders
- Core muscles

INSTRUCTIONS

1. Sit in your chair, in a comfortable position, with your back straight and shoulders relaxed.

2. Place your feet flat on the floor, hip-width apart and maintain a stable posture.

3. Form fists with both hands and bring them up to shoulder height and place them in front of your face.

4. Engage your core muscles for stability.

5. Extend your right arm diagonally across your body in a controlled punch and twist your torso slightly to the left.

6. Return your right fist to the starting position and repeat the motion with your left arm, extending it diagonally across to the right.

7. Continue this alternating cross-punch motion, coordinating with your breath.

8. Exhale as you punch and inhale during the return to the starting position.

9. Keep your pace brisk and controlled during the exercise.

PRECAUTION

Execute the cross punches with control to avoid any sudden or forceful movements.

SEATED SHOULDER SHRUGS

Seated Shoulder Shrugs are a fantastic exercise designed to engage and strengthen the muscles surrounding your shoulders, specifically the trapezius muscles. This seated variation is beneficial for seniors aiming to enhance their shoulder mobility, reduce tension and improve overall upper body function. By incorporating Seated Shoulder Shrugs into your routine, you activate the muscles responsible for elevating your shoulders, promoting better shoulder alignment and relieving stiffness.

Repetitions: 20 repetitions

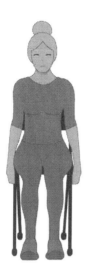 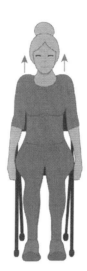 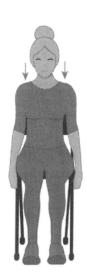

MUSCLES TARGETED

- Trapezius
- Levator scapulae.
- Shoulders
- Upper back

INSTRUCTIONS

1. Comfortably sit in your chair with your back straight and your feet flat on the floor.

2. Deeply inhale the air and lengthen your spine.

3. Exhale as you lift your shoulders towards your ears, engaging the trapezius muscles.

4. Hold the shrugged position for 5-10 seconds, focusing on the contraction in your shoulders.

5. Inhale again as you release the shrug and allow your shoulders to naturally lower.

6. Repeat the movement for 20 repetitions and maintain a slow and controlled pace.

7. Keep your neck and the rest of your body relaxed throughout the exercise, concentrating on the muscles around your shoulders.

PRECAUTION

Shrug the shoulders gently and avoid lifting excessively. If you have shoulder issues, practice the shrugs within a comfortable range.

SEATED CHIN-TO-CHEST STRETCH

The Seated Chin-to-Chest Stretch is a gentle and effective exercise designed to release tension in your neck and upper back. This stretch primarily targets the muscles along the back of your neck and upper spine, helping to alleviate stiffness and promote flexibility. This seated variation is especially beneficial for seniors seeking relief from neck discomfort and aiming to improve their overall neck mobility.

Repetitions: 3 sets of 10 stretches

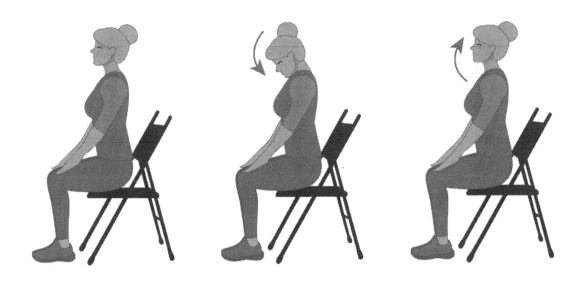

MUSCLES TARGETED

- Sternocleidomastoid
- Neck flexors
- Upper back

INSTRUCTIONS

1. Sit in your chair comfortably with your back straight and your feet flat on the floor.

2. Deeply inhale the air and lengthen your spine.

3. Exhale as you slowly lower your chin towards your chest, feeling a gentle stretch along the back of your neck.

4. Hold the stretched position for 15-30 seconds and allow your neck muscles to relax.

5. Inhale again as you lift your head back to the starting position.

6. Keep your shoulders relaxed and avoid any sudden or forceful movements during the stretch.

PRECAUTION

Stretch the neck gently and avoid overbending. If you have neck concerns, practice the stretch with caution and without strain.

The Only Chair Yoga for Seniors Over 60 Guide You Need

SEATED CROSS-LEGGED FORWARD BEND

Seated Cross-legged Forward Bend is a rejuvenating yoga pose that focuses on enhancing flexibility in the hips and lower back. This seated posture provides a gentle stretch to the muscles while promoting relaxation and mindfulness.

Repetitions: Hold for 45 seconds per side

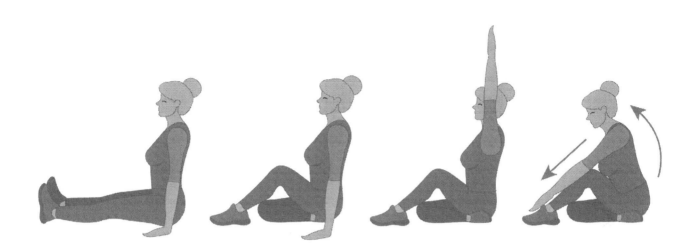

MUSCLES TARGETED

- Hip flexors
- Hamstrings
- Lower back muscles

INSTRUCTIONS

1. Begin by sitting comfortably on the floor with your legs extended straight in front of you.
2. Cross your right leg over your left, place the sole of your right foot on the floor beside your left knee.
3. Bend your left leg and bring your left foot towards your right hip.
4. Ensure both sit bones are grounded on the floor.
5. Inhale and lengthen your spine, sitting tall.
6. As you exhale, gently hinge at your hips, leaning forward over your crossed legs.
7. Reach your hands toward your feet or the floor in front of you and maintain a flat back.
8. Feel the stretch in your right hip and hamstring.
9. Hold your position for 45 seconds, breathing deeply.

PRECAUTION

Be mindful of any discomfort and avoid pushing your body into a position that feels painful. Adjust the intensity of the stretch based on your flexibility.

SEATED KNEE SQUEEZE

Seated Knee Squeeze is a beneficial exercise designed to target the inner thighs and engage the core muscles. This seated movement is particularly effective for improving hip flexibility and strengthening the adductors.

Repetitions: 15 times on each leg

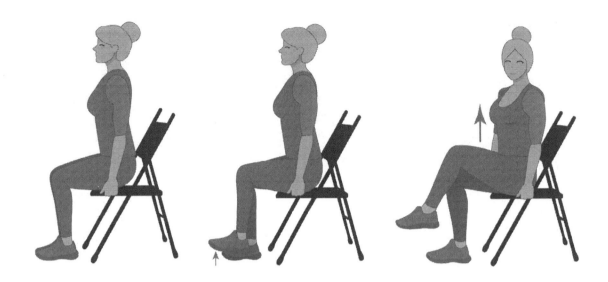

MUSCLES TARGETED

- Adductors (inner thigh muscles)
- Quadriceps
- Core muscles

INSTRUCTIONS

1. Sit in your chair, in a comfortable position, with your back straight and shoulders relaxed.

2. Place your feet flat on the floor, hip-width apart.

3. Engage your core muscles to keep a stable posture.

4. Lift your right foot slightly off the floor, keeping the knee bent.

5. Bring your right knee toward your chest and squeeze the inner thigh muscles.

6. Hold the contraction for a moment, feeling the engagement in the inner thigh.

7. Slowly lower your right foot back to the floor.

8. Repeat the movement on the left side, lift and squeeze the left knee toward your chest.

9. Continue to switch between the right and left legs for a total of 15 repetitions per side.

PRECAUTION

Carry out the knee squeeze movement with controlled and deliberate motions to avoid any sudden or forceful actions.

SEATED CAT-COW STRETCH

The Seated Cat Cow Stretch is a delightful and accessible yoga movement designed to promote spinal flexibility and enhance mobility in the back and shoulders. Tailored for seniors, this seated variation provides a gentle way to experience the fluid motion of the traditional Cat Cow Stretch.

Repetitions: 2 minutes

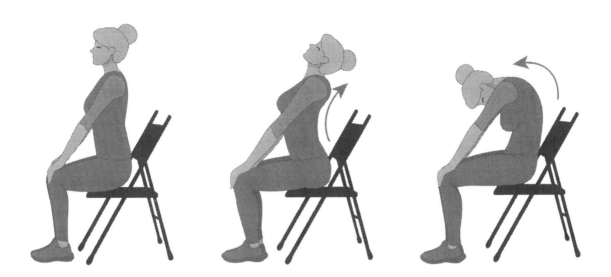

MUSCLES TARGETED

- Spinal erectors
- Abdominal muscles
- Core

INSTRUCTIONS

1. Sit in your chair comfortably with your back straight and feet flat on the floor.

2. Inhale slowly as you arch your back, lift your chest towards the ceiling (Cow position).

3. Exhale as you round your back, tucking your chin towards your chest (Cat position).

4. Repeat the movement, flowing between the Cow and Cat positions, coordinating breath with motion.

5. Continue for 2 minutes and allow the spine to gently flex and extend with each breath.

PRECAUTION

Move with your breath, avoid overarching or rounding your back too much. If you have spine issues, keep the movements gentle.

SEATED BOXER SHUFFLE

Seated Boxer Shuffle is a lively and effective exercise that brings elements of boxing footwork to a seated position. This workout is designed to improve cardiovascular health, leg strength and overall mobility, making it an engaging option for individuals seeking a seated exercise routine with a touch of dynamic movement.

Repetitions: 2-3 sets of 1 minute each

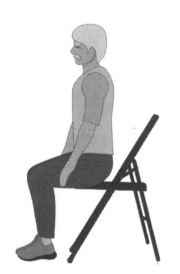 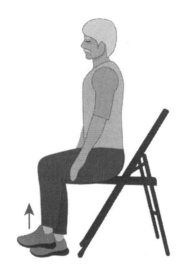 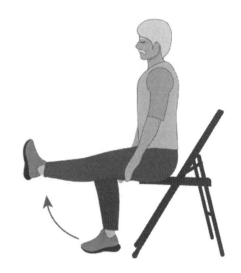

MUSCLES TARGETED

Legs (Quadriceps, Hamstrings, Calves)

Cardiovascular system

Core muscles

INSTRUCTIONS

1. Sit in your chair, in a comfortable position, with your back straight and shoulders relaxed.

2. Place your feet flat on the floor, hip-width apart and maintain a stable and grounded posture.

3. Lift your right foot slightly off the floor and start making small, quick shuffling movements, similar to a boxer's footwork.

4. Alternate the shuffle between your right and left foot and maintain a brisk pace.

5. Engage your core for stability and balance during the shuffle.

6. Coordinate the movement with your breath and maintain a steady rhythm.

7. Feel free to incorporate arm movements, mimicking the motions of a boxer.

8. Continue the seated boxer shuffle for 1 minute, rest briefly and repeat for a total of 3 sets.

PRECAUTION

Carry out the boxer shuffle with controlled and deliberate movements to avoid any sudden or forceful motions.

SEATED FORWARD FOLD (PASCHIMOTTANASANA)

It may indirectly contribute to heart health by reducing stress and improving overall circulation. Incorporating such yoga poses into a well-rounded fitness routine can complement cardiovascular health by fostering relaxation and mental well-being.

Repetitions: 5 times

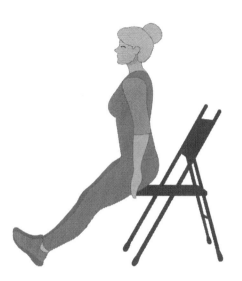
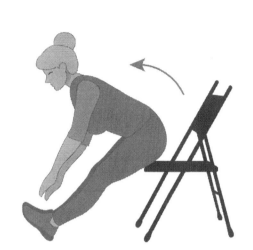

MUSCLES TARGETED

- Hamstrings
- Lower back
- Calves

INSTRUCTIONS

1. Sit on the edge of a chair with your feet together and extended in front of you.

2. Inhale deeply, lengthening your spine and sitting tall.

3. Exhale as you hinge at your hips, leaning forward from your waist toward your toes.

4. Reach your hands toward your feet or shins and maintain a straight spine.

5. Keep your neck in line with your spine, avoiding any strain on your neck.

6. Hold the Seated Forward Fold for 30 seconds to 1 minute, breathing deeply and relaxing into the stretch.

7. Inhale slowly as you slowly lift back to an upright position, using your core muscles.

8. Repeat the forward fold 5 times, gradually increasing the depth of the stretch.

PRECAUTION

Fold forward with a straight back and avoid rounding excessively. If you have spine concerns, practice the fold within your flexibility.

SEATED TWIST (ARDHA MATSYENDRASANA)

Twisting while seated helps maintain spinal flexibility. Hold the back of your chair, gently twist your torso and look over your shoulder. Feel the stretch along your spine. Remember to keep the twist gentle and within a comfortable range. Breathe and release tension.

Repetitions: 5 times

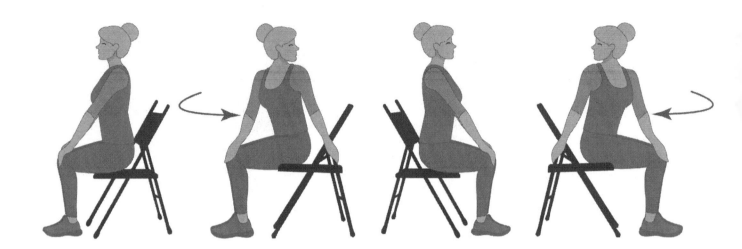

MUSCLES TARGETED

- Obliques
- Spinal rotators.
- Core
- Spine

INSTRUCTIONS

1. Sit in your chair comfortably with your feet flat on the floor and your spine tall.

2. Inhale slowly as you lengthen your spine, sitting tall.

3. Exhale and twist your torso to the right, placing your left hand on your right knee and your right hand on the back of the chair.

4. Inhale to elongate your spine further and exhale to deepen the twist, looking over your right shoulder.

5. Hold the Seated Twist for 20-30 seconds, feeling a gentle stretch in your spine.

6. Inhale slowly as you return to the center and repeat the twist on the other side.

7. Continue to alternate sides, repeating the Seated Twist 5 times per side.

8. Be mindful not to force the twist and listen to your body and maintain a comfortable stretch.

PRECAUTION

Twist the torso gently and avoid over-rotation. If you have spine problems, carry out the twist with control and within a comfortable range.

The Only Chair Yoga for Seniors Over 60 Guide You Need

SEATED LEG LIFTS

Sit with your back straight and lift one leg at a time, engaging your abdominal muscles. This exercise strengthens your core and improves leg strength. Lift your legs at a pace that feels comfortable and remember to breathe. It's a simple yet effective way to keep your lower body active.

Repetitions: 10 times per leg

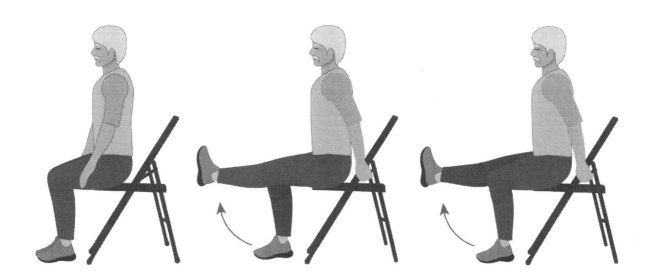

MUSCLES TARGETED

- Quadriceps
- Hip flexors
- Abdominals
- Legs
- Core

INSTRUCTIONS

1. Comfortably sit in your chair with your feet flat on the floor and your back straight.

2. Put your hands on the sides of the chair or your thighs for support.

3. Inhale slowly as you engage your core muscles.

4. Exhale and lift one leg straight out in front of you, keeping it parallel to the floor.

5. Hold the lifted leg for a moment, feeling the contraction in your abdominal muscles.

6. Inhale slowly as you gently lower the leg back down.

7. Repeat the Seated Leg Lifts on the opposite leg.

8. Perform 10 repetitions on each leg, gradually increasing as your strength improves.

PRECAUTION

Raise your legs with control and avoid sudden movements. If you have leg or hip concerns, practice the lifts within your range of motion.

CHAIR RAISED HANDS POSE URDHVA HASTASANA

Bring your hands overhead while seated while reaching for the sky. This pose helps elongate your spine, enhance shoulder flexibility and encourages a sense of openness. Inhale deeply as you lift your arms and feel the stretch along your sides.

Repetitions: 1 minute

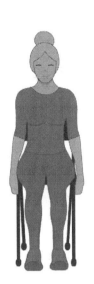 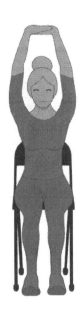 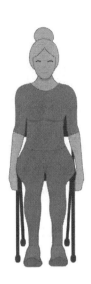

MUSCLES TARGETED

- Deltoids (shoulders)
- Trapezius
- Core
- Shoulders

INSTRUCTIONS

1. Comfortably sit in your chair with your feet flat on the floor and your spine straight.

2. Inhale slowly as you raise your arms overhead while reaching towards the ceiling.

3. Intertwine your fingers and turn your palms upward, extending your arms.

4. Keep your shoulders relaxed and away from your ears.

5. Engage your core muscles and lengthen your spine.

6. Hold the Chair Raised Hands Pose for 20-30 seconds, breathing deeply.

7. Exhale as you lower your arms back down to your sides.

8. Repeat the pose for a few rounds, focusing on the stretch through your arms and the openness in your chest.

PRECAUTION

Raise arms slowly and avoid sudden movements. If you have shoulder concerns, raise your arms within your range of motion.

CHAIR EAGLE – GARUDASANA

Cross one leg over the other and then bring your arms together, as if hugging yourself. This seated eagle pose enhances balance, stretches your upper back and can relieve tension in your shoulders. It's a gentle way to improve flexibility and focus.

Repetitions: 30 seconds

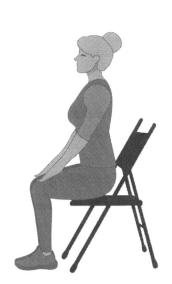
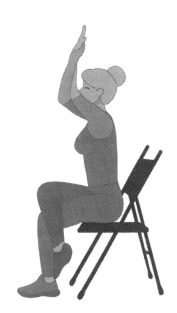

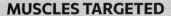
MUSCLES TARGETED

- Hip abductors
- Shoulders
- Trapezius
- Hips
- Shoulders.

INSTRUCTIONS

1. Comfortably sit in your chair with your feet flat on the floor and your spine straight.

2. Cross your right thigh over your left thigh and bring your right foot behind your left calf if possible.

3. Wrap your right foot around your left calf if you can or simply press the foot against the floor.

4. Cross your right arm over your left arm at the elbows and bring your palms together if possible.

5. Lift your elbows slightly and broaden your shoulder blades, feeling a stretch across your upper back.

6. Keep your gaze focused and breathe deeply.

7. Hold the Chair Eagle pose for 30 seconds.

8. Release and repeat on the other side, crossing your left thigh over your right and left arm over right.

PRECAUTION

Cross arms and legs mindfully and avoid over-tightening. If you have joint issues, keep a comfortable cross of limbs.

SEATED ANKLE CIRCLES

While seated, lift your feet off the ground and circle your ankles in both directions. This simple exercise promotes ankle mobility, enhances circulation and can alleviate stiffness. Enjoy the fluid movement and take it at a pace that feels comfortable.

Repetitions: 30 seconds

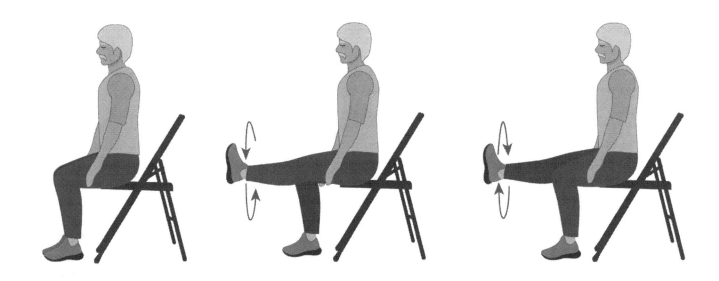

MUSCLES TARGETED

- Ankles
- Calves

INSTRUCTIONS

1. First, sit in your chair in a comfortable position with your feet flat on the floor.
2. Lift your right foot slightly off the ground.
3. Begin to rotate your right ankle in a circular motion, moving clockwise.
4. After several rotations, switch to an anti-clockwise motion.
5. Lower your right foot and repeat the circles with your left ankle.

PRECAUTION

Perform gentle and controlled circles and avoid forceful movements to protect ankle joints.

SEATED KNEE-TO-CHEST LIFTS

Hug one knee at a time toward your chest, alternating between legs. This exercise gently engages your lower abdominal muscles and promotes flexibility in your hips. Breathe steadily and enjoy the soothing effect on your lower back.

Repetitions: 5 lifts per leg

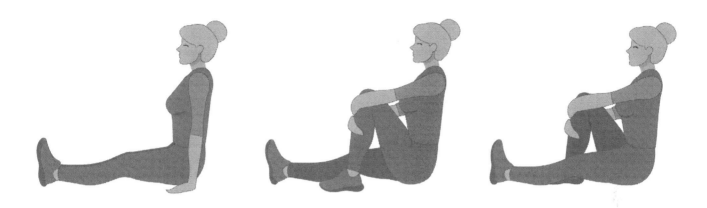

MUSCLES TARGETED

- Hip flexors
- Lower back

INSTRUCTIONS

1. Sit in your chair, in a comfortable position, with your feet flat on the floor.
2. Hold onto the sides of the chair for support.
3. Lift your right knee towards your chest, hugging it with both hands.
4. Hold this position for a moment, feeling a gentle stretch in your lower back and hip.
5. Slowly lower your right foot back to the floor.
6. Repeat the knee-to-chest lift with your left knee.
7. This exercise helps improve hip flexibility and relieve tension in the lower back.

PRECAUTION

Lift knees gradually and if discomfort arises, lower them; keep a smooth motion.

SEATED SHOULDER ROLLS

Lift your shoulders up, roll them back and then down in a circular motion. This exercise helps release tension in your shoulders, improves circulation and promotes shoulder mobility. Move in a way that feels soothing and breathe deeply.

Repetitions: 5 times

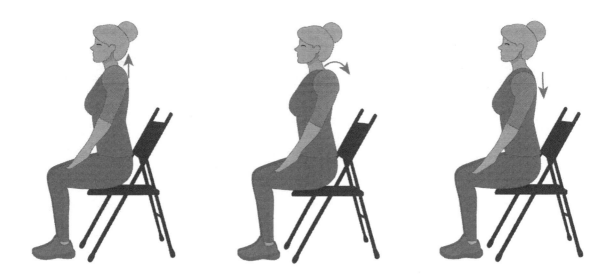

MUSCLES TARGETED

- Shoulders
- Upper back

INSTRUCTIONS

1. Comfortably sit in your chair with your back straight and feet flat on the floor.

2. Relax your arms by your sides.

3. Inhale slowly as you lift your shoulders towards your ears.

4. Exhale and roll your shoulders backward in a circular motion and squeeze your shoulder blades together.

5. Continue the circular motion for 10-15 seconds.

6. Reverse the direction, rolling your shoulders forward for another 10-15 seconds.

7. Repeat the seated shoulder rolls for a total of 5 sets.

8. This exercise helps relieve tension in the shoulders and promotes flexibility.

PRECAUTION

Roll shoulders gently to avoid strain; keep a slow and controlled pace.

SEATED CROSSOVER TOE TOUCHES

Seated Crossover Toe Touches is a seated exercise that combines controlled leg movements with a reaching motion to engage multiple muscle groups and enhance flexibility.

Repetitions: 5 times per side

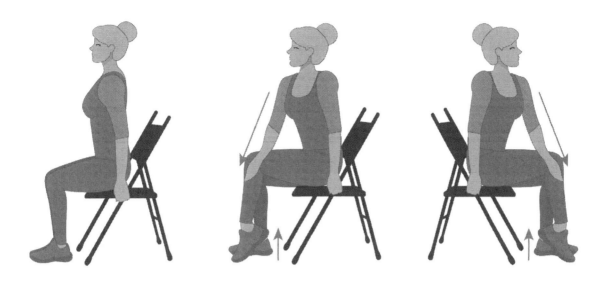

MUSCLES TARGETED

- Hip flexors
- Quadriceps
- Core muscles

INSTRUCTIONS

1. Comfortably, sit in your chair with your back straight and shoulders relaxed.

2. Keep your feet flat on the floor, maintaining hip-width apart.

3. Lift your right knee toward your chest while keeping your foot on the ground.

4. As you lower your right foot, reach across your body with your left hand to touch the outside of your right foot.

5. Return to the starting position and repeat the motion on the other side, lifting the left knee and reaching with the right hand.

6. Continue this crossover toe-touching motion, alternating between legs and reaching across your body.

7. Coordinate the movement with your breath, inhaling as you lift and exhaling as you reach.

PRECAUTION

Practice this exercise with smooth, controlled movements, avoiding sudden or forceful actions. If you experience any discomfort, adjust the intensity or range of motion as needed.

SEATED WRIST STRETCHES

Extend your arms forward, flex and extend your wrists and then circle them in both directions. This seated exercise is beneficial for maintaining wrist flexibility and preventing stiffness. Take your time and enjoy the rejuvenating movement.

Repetitions: 10 times per wrist

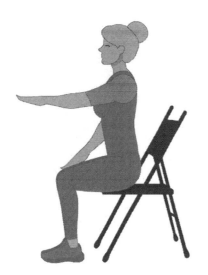 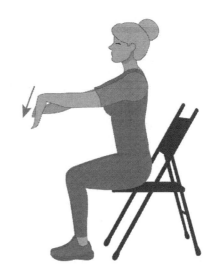

MUSCLES TARGETED

- Wrists
- Forearms

INSTRUCTIONS

1. Comfortably sit in your chair with your back straight and feet flat on the floor.

2. Extend your right arm straight out with the palm facing down.

3. Use your left hand to gently press down on the fingers of your right hand, feeling a stretch in the wrist and forearm.

4. Hold the stretch for 15-20 seconds.

5. Switch to the left hand, extending the arm and pressing down with the right hand.

PRECAUTION

Stretch wrists gently; stop if you feel any sharp pain or discomfort.

The Only Chair Yoga for Seniors Over 60 Guide You Need

SEATED ELBOW CIRCLES

Gently rotate your elbows in circular motions while seated. This exercise helps improve elbow flexibility, reduce stiffness and promotes better circulation in the arms. Move your elbows clockwise and counterclockwise, enjoying the soothing effect on your joints.

Repetitions: 10 times per elbow

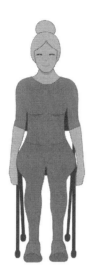 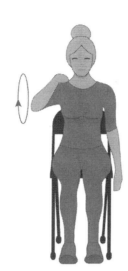 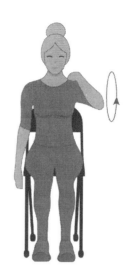

MUSCLES TARGETED

- Elbows
- Forearms

INSTRUCTIONS

1. Sit in your chair comfortably with your back straight and feet flat on the floor.

2. Lift your right arm, bending it at the elbow and make small circular motions with your elbow.

3. Rotate the elbow clockwise for 10-15 seconds.

4. Reverse the direction, making anticlockwise circles for another 10-15 seconds.

5. Lower your right arm and repeat the circles with your left elbow.

PRECAUTION

Circle elbows smoothly; if you experience discomfort, reduce the range of motion.

28-DAY BEGINNER CHALLENGE

WEEK 01

Days	Warm-Up	Heart Health	Bad posture	Weight-loss	Joint Mobility
Monday	Seated Marching **p.13**	Upward Salute Pose **p.17**	Seated Shoulder Shrugs **p.23**	Seated Boxer Shuffle **p.28**	Seated Shoulder Rolls **p.36**
Tuesday	Seated Arm Reaches **p.14**	Seated Butterfly Stretch **p.18**	Seated Chin-To-Chest Stretch **p.24**	Seated Forward Fold (Paschimottanasana) **p.29**	Seated Crossover Toe Touches **p.37**
Wednesday	Seated High Knees **p.15**	Bow Pose **p.19**	Seated Cross-Legged Forward Bend **p.25**	Seated Twist (Ardha Matsyendrasana) **p.30**	Seated Wrist Stretches **p.38**
Thursday	Forward Fold (Uttanasana) **p.16**	Seated Shoulder Opener **p.20**	Seated Knee Squeeze **p.26**	Seated Leg Lifts **p.31**	Seated Elbow Circles **p.39**
Friday	Seated Marching **p.13**	Seated Sunflower Stretch **p.21**	Seated Cat-Cow Stretch **p.27**	Chair Raised Hands Pose Urdhva Hastasana **p.32**	Seated Shoulder Rolls **p.36**
Saturday	Seated Arm Reaches **p.14**	Seated Cross Punches **p.22**	Seated Chin-To-Chest Stretch **p.24**	Chair Eagle – Garudasana **p.33**	Seated Crossover Toe Touches **p.37**
Sunday	Seated High Knees **p.15**	Bow Pose **p.19**	Seated Cross-Legged Forward Bend **p.25**	Seated Boxer Shuffle **p.28**	Seated Wrist Stretches **p.38**

WEEK 02

Days	Warm-Up	Heart Health	Bad posture	Weight-loss	Joint Mobility
Monday	Forward Fold (Uttanasana) **p.16**	Upward Salute Pose **p.17**	Seated Cross-Legged Forward Bend **p.25**	Seated Forward Fold (Paschimotta-nasana) **p.29**	Seated Shoulder Rolls **p.36**
Tuesday	Seated Marching **p.13**	Seated Butterfly Stretch **p.18**	Seated Knee Squeeze **p.26**	Seated Twist (Ardha Matsy-endrasana) **p.30**	Seated Cross-over Toe Touches **p.37**
Wednes-day	Seated Arm Reaches **p.14**	Bow Pose **p.19**	Seated Cat-Cow Stretch **p.27**	Seated Leg Lifts **p.31**	Seated Wrist Stretches **p.38**
Thursday	Seated March-ing **p.13**	Seated Shoulder Opener **p.20**	Seated Shoulder Shrugs **p.23**	Chair Raised Hands Pose Urdhva Hastasana **p.32**	Seated Elbow Circles **p.39**
Friday	Seated Arm Reaches **p.14**	Seated Sunflower Stretch **p.21**	Seated Chin-To-Chest Stretch **p.24**	Chair Eagle – Garudasana **p.33**	Seated Shoulder Rolls **p.36**
Saturday	Seated High Knees **p.15**	Seated Cross Punches **p.22**	Seated Cross-Legged Forward Bend **p.25**	Seated Forward Fold (Paschimotta-nasana) **p.29**	Seated Cross-over Toe Touches **p.37**
Sunday	Forward Fold (Uttanasana) **p.16**	Seated Shoulder Opener **p.20**	Seated Knee Squeeze **p.26**	Seated Twist (Ardha Matsy-endrasana) **p.30**	Seated Wrist Stretches **p.38**

WEEK 03

Days	Warm-Up	Heart Health	Bad posture	Weight-loss	Joint Mobility
Monday	Seated Marching **p.13**	Upward Salute Pose **p.17**	Seated Shoulder Shrugs **p.23**	Seated Boxer Shuffle **p.28**	Seated Shoulder Rolls **p.36**
Tuesday	Seated Arm Reaches **p.14**	Seated Butterfly Stretch **p.18**	Seated Chin-To-Chest Stretch **p.24**	Seated Forward Fold (Paschimottanasana) **p.29**	Seated Crossover Toe Touches **p.37**
Wednesday	Seated High Knees **p.15**	Bow Pose **p.19**	Seated Cross-Legged Forward Bend **p.25**	Seated Twist (Ardha Matsyendrasana) **p.30**	Seated Wrist Stretches **p.38**
Thursday	Forward Fold (Uttanasana) **p.16**	Seated Shoulder Opener **p.20**	Seated Knee Squeeze **p.26**	Seated Leg Lifts **p.31**	Seated Shoulder Rolls **p.36**
Friday	Seated Marching **p.13**	Seated Sunflower Stretch **p.21**	Seated Cat-Cow Stretch **p.27**	Chair Raised Hands Pose Urdhva Hastasana **p.32**	Seated Crossover Toe Touches **p.37**
Saturday	Seated Arm Reaches **p.14**	Seated Cross Punches **p.22**	Seated Shoulder Shrugs **p.23**	Chair Eagle – Garudasana **p.33**	Seated Wrist Stretches **p.38**
Sunday	Seated High Knees **p.15**	Seated Butterfly Stretch **p.18**	Seated Chin-To-Chest Stretch **p.24**	Seated Boxer Shuffle **p.28**	Seated Elbow Circles **p.39**

WEEK 04

Days	Warm-Up	Heart Health	Bad posture	Weight-loss	Joint Mobility
Monday	Forward Fold (Uttanasana) **p.16**	Bow Pose **p.19**	Seated Cross-Legged Forward Bend **p.25**	Seated Forward Fold (Paschimotta-nasana) **p.29**	Seated Shoulder Rolls **p.36**
Tuesday	Seated Marching **p.13**	Seated Butterfly Stretch **p.18**	Seated Knee Squeeze **p.26**	Seated Twist (Ardha Matsyendrasana) **p.30**	Seated Crossover Toe Touches **p.37**
Wednesday	Seated Arm Reaches **p.14**	Bow Pose **p.19**	Seated Cat-Cow Stretch **p.27**	Seated Leg Lifts **p.31**	Seated Wrist Stretches **p.38**
Thursday	Seated Marching **p.13**	Seated Shoulder Opener **p.20**	Seated Shoulder Shrugs **p.23**	Chair Raised Hands Pose Urdhva Hastasana **p.32**	Seated Elbow Circles **p.39**
Friday	Seated Arm Reaches **p.14**	Seated Sunflower Stretch **p.21**	Seated Chin-To-Chest Stretch **p.24**	Chair Eagle – Garudasana **p.33**	Seated Shoulder Rolls **p.36**
Saturday	Seated High Knees **p.15**	Seated Cross Punches **p.22**	Seated Cross-Legged Forward Bend **p.25**	Seated Forward Fold (Paschimotta-nasana) **p.29**	Seated Crossover Toe Touches **p.37**
Sunday	Forward Fold (Uttanasana) **p.16**	Seated Shoulder Opener **p.20**	Seated Knee Squeeze **p.26**	Seated Twist (Ardha Matsyendrasana) **p.30**	Seated Wrist Stretches **p.38**

CHAPTER 4:
PROGRESSING INTO DEPER POSES

POSES TO WARM-UP

SEATED SIDE LEG LIFTS

Seated Side Leg Lifts are an excellent exercise to target the outer thighs and hip abductors while promoting core stability. This seated variation is suitable for individuals of various fitness levels and can be especially beneficial for those looking to improve hip strength and mobility.

Repetitions: 3 sets of 12 lifts per side

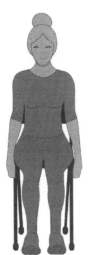 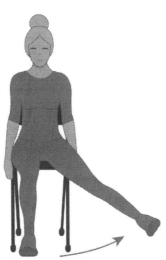 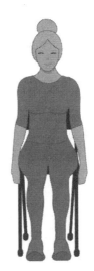 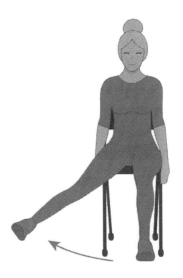

MUSCLES TARGETED

- Outer thighs (Hip abductors)
- Quadriceps
- Core muscles

INSTRUCTIONS

1. Comfortably sit in your chair with your back straight and shoulders relaxed.

2. Place your feet flat on the floor and maintain a hip-width distance between them.

3. Engage your core muscles to stabilize your torso.

4. Lift your right leg out to the side, keeping it straight and pause at the highest point.

5. Lower your right leg back to the starting position.

6. Repeat the motion with your left leg and lift it to the side and holding for a moment.

7. In an alternate movement, switch between right and left leg lifts for a set of 12per side.

8. Coordinate the leg lifts with your breath, exhaling as you lift and inhaling as you lower.

9. Perform three sets, taking short breaks between sets.

PRECAUTION

Do the leg lifts with controlled movements to avoid any strain or injury.

If you have any hip or knee issues, limit the range of motion to a point that is comfortable for you.

CHAIR TAP DANCE

Chair Tap Dance is a delightful and creative exercise designed for seniors to improve lower body strength, coordination and balance. This seated activity mimics the rhythmic motion of tap dancing while sitting comfortably in a chair.

Repetitions: 90 seconds

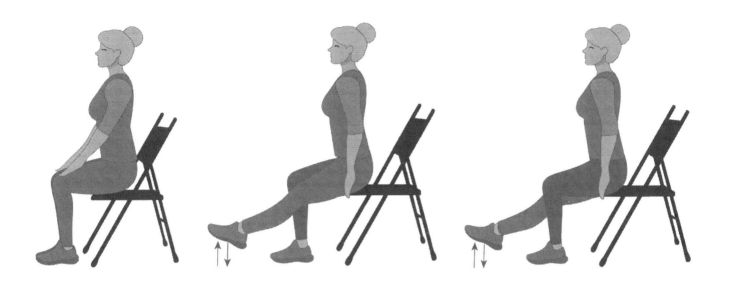

MUSCLES TARGETED

- Quadriceps
- Hamstrings
- Calf muscles

INSTRUCTIONS

1. Sit in a sturdy chair with your back straight and feet flat on the floor.

2. Lift your right foot slightly off the floor and tap it gently on the ground in front of you.

3. Bring your right foot back to the starting position and repeat the tapping motion with your left foot.

4. Continue to switch the tapping motion between your right and left feet.

5. Add variation by tapping to the sides, behind or creating a rhythmic pattern.

6. Engage your arms by tapping your hands on your thighs or the sides of the chair to add flair to the dance.

7. Coordinate your tapping with the beat of your favorite music for an enjoyable experience.

PRECAUTION

Keep movements light and avoid high impact and excessive force on your joints.

SEATED ROWING

Seated Rowing is an effective exercise that targets the muscles of the upper back, shoulders and arms while promoting good posture. This seated variation provides a low-impact option for individuals seeking to improve their upper body strength and endurance.

Repetitions: 3 sets of 12 rows

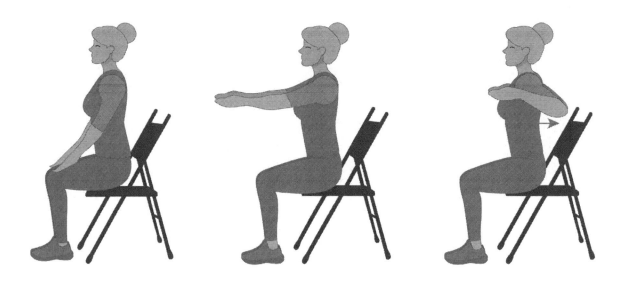

MUSCLES TARGETED

- Rhomboids
- Trapezius
- Lats (Latissimus dorsi)
- Biceps

INSTRUCTIONS

1. First, sit in your chair in a comfortable position with your back straight, shoulders relaxed and feet flat on the floor.

2. Extend your arms straight in front of you, parallel to the ground, palms facing each other.

3. Engage your core muscles to maintain stability.

4. Pull your elbows back and squeeze your shoulder blades together as you bring your hands toward your chest.

5. Keep your wrists straight and close to your body during the movement.

6. Extend your arms back to the starting position and maintain control.

PRECAUTION

Carry out the seated rowing exercise with controlled movements to avoid strain or injury.

If you have any preexisting back issues, consult with a healthcare professional before attempting this exercise. Maintain proper posture throughout the exercise to maximize its benefits.

SEATED BICYCLE CRUNCHES

Seated Bicycle Crunches offer an effective seated variation of the traditional bicycle crunch exercise, engaging the core muscles while providing a low-impact option for individuals with mobility limitations. This exercise is beneficial for strengthening the abdominal muscles and improving overall core stability.

Repetitions: 3 sets of 15 crunches (alternating sides)

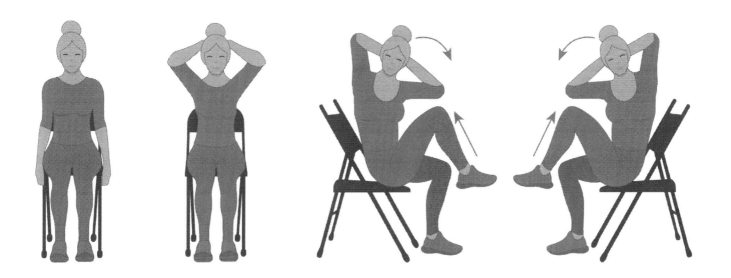

MUSCLES TARGETED

- Rectus abdominis
- Obliques
- Hip flexors

INSTRUCTIONS

1. Sit in your chair comfortably with your back straight and shoulders relaxed.
2. Place your feet flat on the floor, hip-width apart.
3. Put your hands behind your head, elbows pointing outward.
4. Lift your right knee toward your chest while simultaneously twisting your torso to bring your left elbow toward the right knee.
5. Extend your right leg straight while bringing your left knee toward your chest and twisting your torso to bring your right elbow toward the left knee.
6. Continue this alternating motion, mimicking a bicycling motion with your legs while twisting your torso.
7. Coordinate the movement with your breath, exhaling as you twist and inhaling as you return to the starting position.
8. Perform 15 bicycle crunches, alternating sides.
9. Complete three sets, taking short breaks between sets.

PRECAUTION

Carry out the bicycle crunches with controlled and deliberate movements to avoid strain. If you have any preexisting back issues, consult with a healthcare professional before attempting this exercise.

SEATED SIDE LEG CROSS

Seated Side Leg Cross is an effective exercise that targets the outer thighs and hip abductors while promoting core engagement. This seated variation is suitable for individuals of various fitness levels and can be particularly beneficial for those looking to enhance hip strength and flexibility.

Repetitions: 3 sets of 12 crosses per side

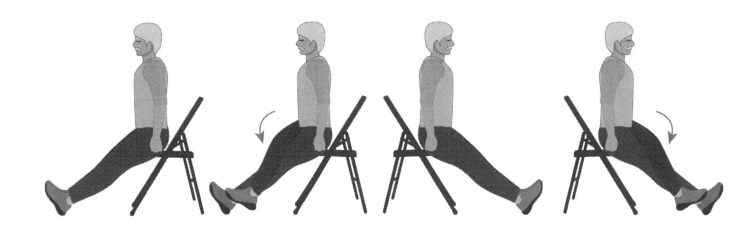

MUSCLES TARGETED

- Outer thighs (Hip abductors)
- Quadriceps
- Core muscles

INSTRUCTIONS

1. First, sit in your chair in a comfortable position with your back straight and shoulders relaxed.

2. Place your feet flat on the floor and maintain a hip-width distance between them.

3. Engage your core muscles to stabilize your torso.

4. Lift your right leg and cross it over your left leg, creating an X shape with your thighs.

5. Return your right foot to the floor and then lift your left leg, crossing it over your right leg.

6. In an alternate movement, switch between right and left leg crosses for a set of 12 per side.

7. Coordinate the leg crosses with your breath, exhaling as you lift and inhaling as you lower.

8. Perform three sets, taking short breaks between sets.

PRECAUTION

Do the leg crosses with controlled movements to avoid any strain or injury. If you have any hip or knee issues, limit the range of motion to a point that is comfortable for you. Maintain proper posture throughout the exercise to maximize its effectiveness.

SEATED SIDE LEG RAISES

Seated Side Leg Raises are a beneficial exercise focusing on strengthening the outer hip and thigh muscles while providing a seated alternative for individuals with varying fitness levels. This exercise is particularly effective for enhancing hip mobility and toning the muscles along the side of the leg.

Repetitions: 3 sets of 15 raises per side

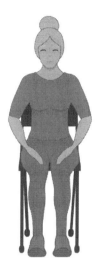 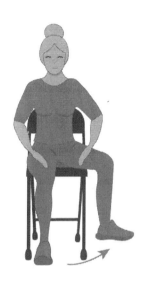 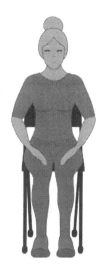 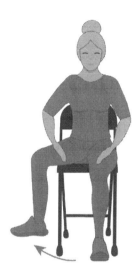

MUSCLES TARGETED

- Abductors (outer hip muscles)
- Quadriceps
- Core muscles

INSTRUCTIONS

1. First, sit in your chair in a comfortable position with your back straight and shoulders relaxed.

2. Place your feet flat on the floor and maintain a hip-width distance between them.

3. Keep your hands resting on your thighs or hold onto the sides of the chair for support.

4. Lift your right leg to the side and make sure that your foot remains parallel to the floor.

5. Lower your right leg back to the starting position.

6. Repeat the side leg raise with your right leg for 15 repetitions.

7. Switch to your left leg and lift it to the side and back down.

8. Continue to switch between right and left side leg raises for a total of 3 sets.

9. Coordinate the raises with your breath, exhaling as you lift and inhaling as you lower.

10. Take short breaks between sets.

PRECAUTION

Do the side leg raises with controlled movements to avoid any strain or injury.

If you experience discomfort, reduce the range of motion or use additional support.

SEATED CHEST EXPANSION

Seated Chest Expansion is a beneficial exercise that targets the muscles in the chest and shoulders, promoting better posture and flexibility. This seated variation is particularly suitable for individuals who may have difficulty with standing exercises or those looking to enhance upper body mobility while seated.

Repetitions: 3 sets of 12 expansions

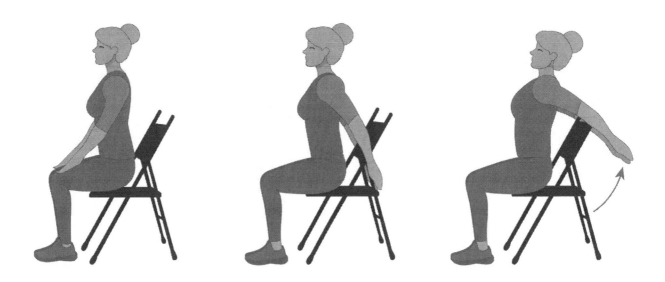

MUSCLES TARGETED

- Chest muscles (Pectoralis major)
- Shoulder muscles (Deltoids)
- Upper back muscles (Rhomboids)

INSTRUCTIONS

1. Comfortably sit in your chair with your back straight and shoulders relaxed.

2. Place your feet flat on the floor and maintain a hip-width distance between them.

3. Intertwine your fingers and bring your hands behind your back, straightening your arms.

4. Inhale slowly as you lift your arms slightly away from your back, opening up your chest.

5. Exhale and gently squeeze your shoulder blades together, emphasizing the chest expansion.

6. Hold this expanded position for a moment, feeling a stretch across your chest and shoulders.

7. Inhale slowly as you release the expansion and bring your arms back down.

8. Take short breaks between sets.

PRECAUTION

Practice the chest expansions with controlled movements to avoid any strain or injury.

If you experience discomfort, reduce the range of motion or use additional support.

SEATED QUADRICEPS STRETCH

Seated Quadriceps Stretch is a gentle and effective exercise designed to improve flexibility in the quadriceps muscles, which are located at the front of your thighs. This seated variation is particularly suitable for individuals who may have difficulty with standing stretches or those looking to enhance quadriceps mobility while seated.

Repetitions: 3 sets of 15 seconds stretch on each leg

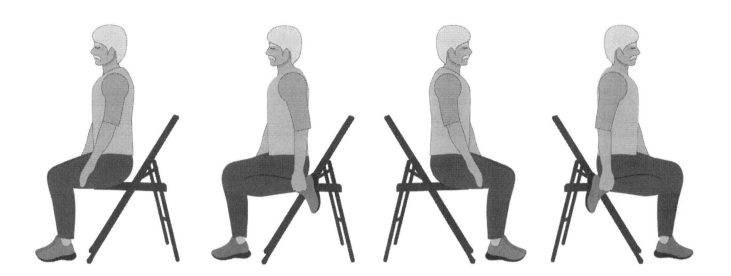

MUSCLES TARGETED

- Quadriceps muscles
- Hip flexors
- Core muscles

INSTRUCTIONS

1. First, sit in your chair in a comfortable position with your back straight and shoulders relaxed.
2. Place your feet flat on the floor, hip-width apart.
3. Lift your right foot, bending your knee and bring it towards your buttocks.
4. Reach behind you with your right hand and gently grasp your right ankle.
5. Keep your back straight and ensure both knees are close together.
6. Feel the stretch in the front of your right thigh and hip.
7. Hold the stretch for 15 seconds, focusing on breathing deeply and relaxing into the stretch.
8. Release your right ankle and lower your right foot back to the floor.
9. Repeat the stretch on your left leg, following the same instructions.
10. In an alternate movement, switch between right and left leg stretches for a total of 3 sets.
11. Take short breaks between sets.

PRECAUTION

Do the quadriceps stretch with controlled movements to avoid any strain or injury. If you experience discomfort, reduce the range of motion or use additional support.

SEATED PRAYER TWIST

Seated Prayer Twist is a beneficial seated exercise that targets the muscles in the core, spine and shoulders. This exercise helps improve spinal mobility and promotes a gentle stretch through the torso. It's a suitable option for individuals who may have difficulty with standing or floor-based twists.

Repetitions: 3 sets of 8 twists per side

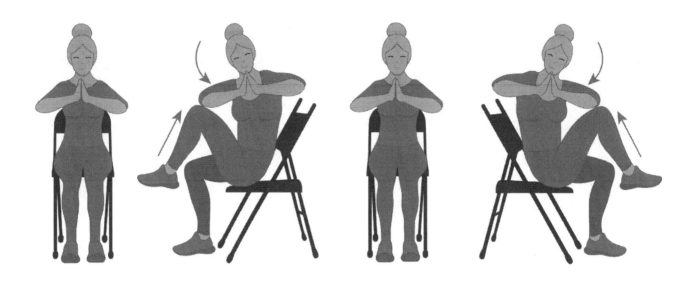

MUSCLES TARGETED

- Abdominal muscles (Obliques)
- Spinal muscles
- Shoulder muscles

INSTRUCTIONS

1. Sit in your chair, in a comfortable position, with your back straight and shoulders relaxed.
2. Place your feet flat on the floor, hip-width apart.
3. Keep your knees together and your hands in a prayer position in front of your chest.
4. Inhale slowly as you lengthen your spine and twist your torso to the right and bring your left elbow to the outside of your right knee.
5. Exhale and engage your core as you deepen the twist, feeling a gentle stretch along your spine.
6. Hold the twist for a moment and maintain a tall and lifted posture.

7. Inhale and return to the center and bring your hands back to the prayer position.
8. Repeat the twist, this time to the left and bring your right elbow to the outside of your left knee.
9. Exhale, deepen the twist and hold for a moment.
10. Return to the center and continue to switch twists for a total of 3 sets per side.
11. Take short breaks between sets.

PRECAUTION

Practice the seated prayer twist with controlled movements to avoid any strain or injury. If you experience discomfort, reduce the range of motion or use additional support. Avoid forcing the twist; move within a comfortable range for your body.

SEATED LATERAL ARM RAISES

Seated Lateral Arm Raises are a simple yet effective seated exercise designed to strengthen the shoulder muscles. This exercise is particularly beneficial for seniors or individuals who may have difficulty standing for prolonged periods. By incorporating lateral arm raises into a seated routine, one can enhance upper body strength and flexibility.

Repetitions: 3 sets of 20 raises

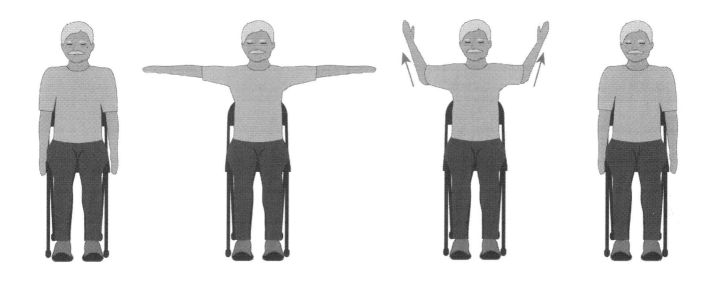

MUSCLES TARGETED

- Deltoids (Shoulder muscles)
- Upper back muscles
- Triceps (Back of the arms)

INSTRUCTIONS

1. Sit in your chair comfortably with your back straight and shoulders relaxed.

2. Place your feet flat on the floor, hip-width apart.

3. Keep your arms by your sides, palms facing inward.

4. Inhale and raise both arms laterally to shoulder height and maintain a slight bend in the elbows.

5. Hold the raised position for a moment, engaging the shoulder muscles.

6. Exhale as you lower your arms back to the starting position by your sides.

7. Repeat the motion for the recommended number of repetitions.

8. Coordinate the movement with your breath, inhaling as you raise your arms and exhaling as you lower them.

9. Take short breaks between sets.

PRECAUTION

Avoid any jerky or sudden movements while raising or lowering your arms.

Start with light weights or no weights at all, gradually increasing resistance as your strength improves.

SEATED BALANCE POSE WITH ARM REACH

Seated Balance Pose with Arm Reach is a seated yoga variation that enhances stability, core strength and upper body flexibility. This gentle exercise is well-suited for seniors, offering a combination of balance and arm-reaching movements.

Repetitions: 2 minutes

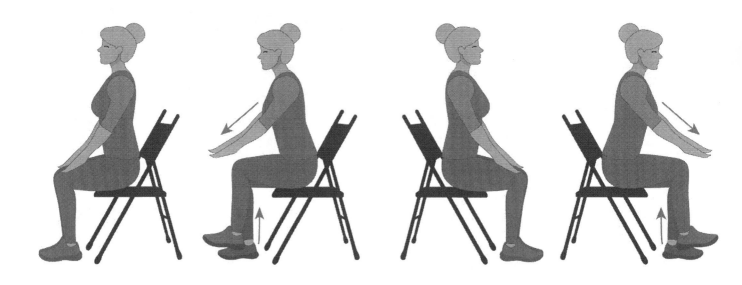

MUSCLES TARGETED

- Hip flexors
- Quadriceps
- Core muscles
- Shoulders and arms

INSTRUCTIONS

1. Comfortably sit in your chair with your back straight and shoulders relaxed.

2. Place your feet flat on the floor and maintain hip-width apart.

3. Lift your right knee toward your chest, finding a comfortable height.

4. Simultaneously extend both arms forward while reaching toward your lifted knee.

5. Hold the balance for a few breaths, engaging your core muscles to stabilize.

6. Lower your right foot back to the floor and return your arms to the starting position.

7. Repeat the sequence with your left knee and lift it towards your chest while reaching your arms forward.

PRECAUTION

Lift your knees gently to avoid any sudden or forceful movements.

SEATED LEG CROSS TOE TOUCHES

Seated Leg Cross Toe Touches offer seniors a targeted exercise to enhance flexibility and engage the core muscles. This seated routine promotes overall lower body strength and helps maintain mobility.

Repetitions: 8 times per leg

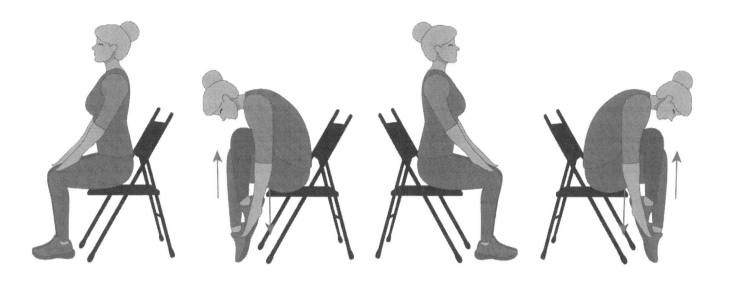

MUSCLES TARGETED

- Hip flexors
- Quadriceps
- Core muscles

INSTRUCTIONS

1. Comfortably, sit in your chair with your back straight and shoulders relaxed.

2. Keep your feet flat on the floor, maintaining hip-width apart.

3. Lift your right knee toward your chest, crossing it over your left leg.

4. Extend your arms towards your right foot, reaching for a toe touch.

5. Slowly return to the starting position, lowering your right foot to the floor.

6. Repeat the motion on the opposite side, lifting your left knee and reaching for your left foot.

7. Continue alternating between right and left, performing leg cross-toe touches with control.

8. Coordinate the movement with your breath, exhaling as you reach and inhaling as you lower.

PRECAUTION

Execute Seated Leg Cross Toe Touches cautiously. Keep a gentle stretch and avoid any abrupt or forceful movements.

SEATED SIDE BEND

The Seated Side Bend is a wonderful exercise designed to enhance flexibility and stretch the muscles along your sides, particularly the obliques. This seated variation is perfect for seniors looking to improve their lateral mobility and posture. Incorporating the Seated Side Bend into your routine provides a gentle yet effective stretch, promoting better range of motion in the torso.

Repetitions: 3 sets of 10 bends per side

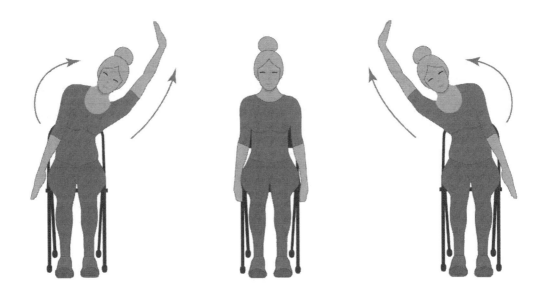

MUSCLES TARGETED

- Internal and external obliques
- Quadratus lumborum
- Waist, sides

INSTRUCTIONS

1. First, sit in your chair in a comfortable position with your back straight and your feet flat on the floor.
2. Deeply inhale the air and lengthen your spine.
3. Exhale as you gently lean to one side and bring your arm overhead and reach toward the opposite side.
4. Hold the stretched position for 15-30 seconds, feeling a gentle stretch along your side.
5. Inhale again as you return to the upright position.
6. Repeat the movement on the other side, leaning and reaching in the opposite direction.
7. Continue to switch sides for 3 sets and maintain a slow and controlled pace.

PRECAUTION

Bend to the side slowly and avoid overstretching. If you have spine concerns, practice the movement within your comfort range.

SEATED CACTUS ARMS

The Seated Cactus Arms exercise is a wonderful way to open up your chest, improve shoulder mobility and counteract the effects of slouching or sitting for extended periods. This seated variation is especially beneficial for seniors looking to enhance their upper body flexibility.

Repetitions: 1 minute

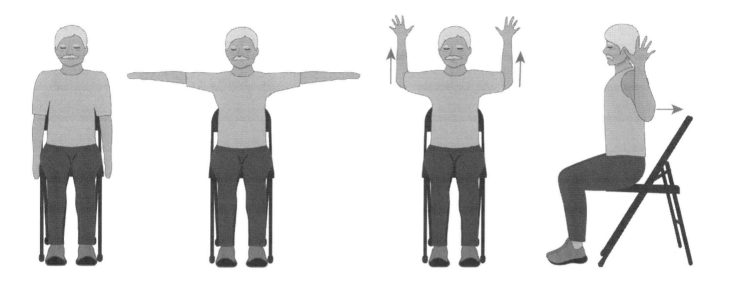

MUSCLES TARGETED

- Deltoids (shoulders)
- Trapezius
- Rhomboids
- Shoulders
- Upper back

INSTRUCTIONS

1. First, sit in your chair in a comfortable position with your back straight and your feet flat on the floor.

2. Lift your arms to shoulder height, bending them at the elbows to create a 90-degree angle.

3. Open your palms, spreading your fingers wide, resembling a cactus shape.

4. Inhale deeply as you squeeze your shoulder blades together and bring your elbows back.

5. Hold this position for 10-15 seconds, feeling a gentle stretch across your chest.

6. Exhale as you release the arms back to the starting position.

7. Repeat the movement for 2-3 sets and maintain a slow and controlled pace.

PRECAUTION

Open your arms slowly and avoid overstretching. If you have shoulder issues, practice the movement within your comfort zone.

SEATED WALL ANGELS

Seated Wall Angels is a fantastic exercise that targets multiple muscle groups, making it an excellent choice for seniors aiming to improve their upper body strength and flexibility. This seated variation is gentle yet effective, focusing on the shoulders, upper back and arms.

Repetitions: 15 times

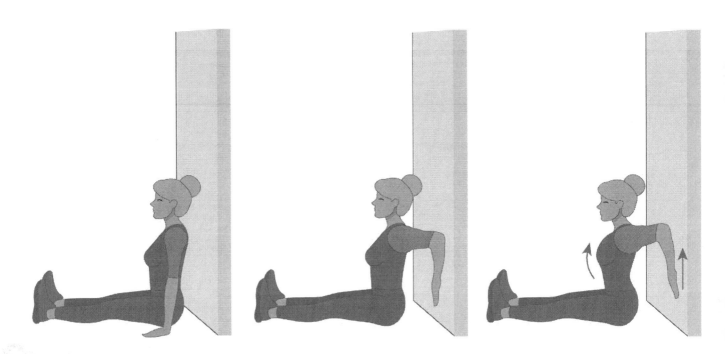

MUSCLES TARGETED

- Rhomboids
- Deltoids (shoulders)
- Trapezius
- Upper back
- Shoulders

INSTRUCTIONS

1. Sit against a wall with your back straight and your feet flat on the floor.

2. Place your arms against the wall and form a goalpost shape with your elbows at a 90-degree angle.

3. Inhale deeply as you slide your arms up the wall, keeping your elbows and wrists in contact with the surface.

4. As you reach upward, focus on squeezing your shoulder blades together and opening your chest.

5. Exhale as you slowly lower your arms back down to the starting position.

6. Pay attention to your posture and make sure that your back stays in contact with the wall throughout the exercise.

PRECAUTION

Keep your back against the wall and avoid arching. If you have shoulder or neck problems, perform smaller movements.

SEATED CROSS-LEGGED ARM TWIST

Seated Cross-Legged Arm Twist is a seated exercise designed to enhance mobility and flexibility in the upper body while providing a gentle workout for the core muscles. Tailored for individuals seeking a low-impact routine, this exercise engages the hip flexors, quadriceps and core muscles.

Repetitions: 30 seconds

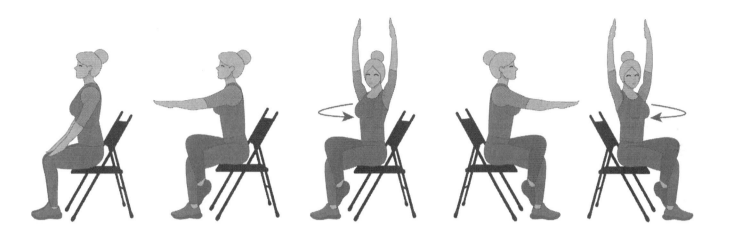

MUSCLES TARGETED

- Hip flexors
- Quadriceps
- Core muscles

INSTRUCTIONS

1. First, sit in your chair in a comfortable position with your back straight and shoulders relaxed.

2. Place your feet flat on the floor, hip-width apart.

3. Cross your right leg over your left leg and form a comfortable cross-legged position.

4. Extend your arms straight out in front of you at shoulder height, parallel to the floor.

5. Inhale deeply as you twist your torso to the right and bring your arms along with the movement.

6. Exhale and return to the center.

7. Repeat the twist to the left side, inhaling as you twist and exhaling as you return to the center.

8. In an alternate movement, switch between right and left twists, coordinating the movement with your breath.

PRECAUTION

Practice the seated cross-legged arm twist with smooth and controlled motions.

SEATED WARRIOR II

Bring the strength of a warrior into your seated position. Extend your arms, stretch them wide and feel the engagement in your upper body. This exercise helps maintain arm strength and shoulder flexibility. Breathe deeply and enjoy the empowering feeling of the seated warrior.

Repetitions: 1 minute

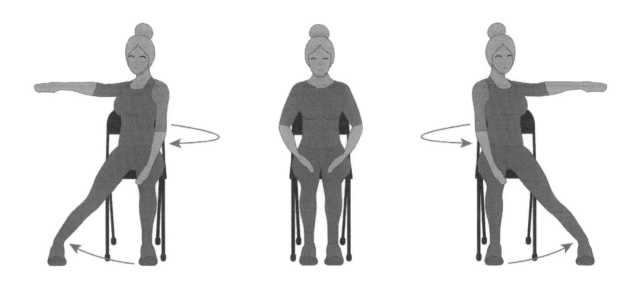

MUSCLES TARGETED

- Quadriceps
- Hip abductors
- Deltoids (shoulders).
- Legs
- Shoulders

INSTRUCTIONS

1. Comfortably sit in your chair with your feet flat on the floor and your back straight.

2. Extend your right leg straight out to the side, keeping your foot on the floor.

3. Turn your torso to the right and bring your left hand to rest on your left thigh.

4. Extend your right arm straight out to the side, parallel to the floor, with your palm facing down.

5. Engage your core muscles and open your chest to face the right side.

6. Hold the Seated Warrior II for 20-30 seconds, breathing deeply.

7. Return to the center and switch to the opposite side, extending the left leg and turning your torso to the left.

8. Repeat the Seated Warrior II on both sides for a balanced stretch.

PRECAUTION

Open the arms and legs gently and avoid over-stretching. If you have hip or shoulder problems, keep a comfortable stance.

SEATED SUN SALUTATION (SURYA NAMASKAR)

Adapted for a seated position, this sun salutation involves gentle movements to warm up your body. Raise your arms overhead, fold forward and stretch out your spine. It's a revitalizing sequence that promotes circulation and flexibility while seated comfortably. Take it at your own pace and enjoy the energizing flow.

Repetitions: 1 minute

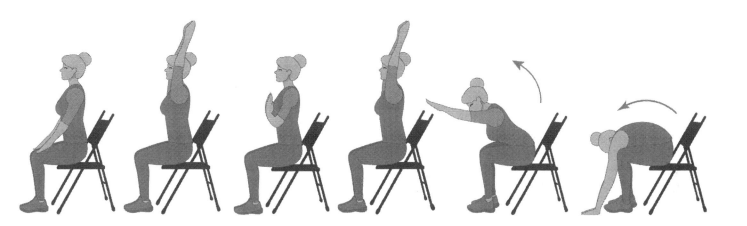

MUSCLES TARGETED

- Core
- Arms
- Legs
- Total body

INSTRUCTIONS

1. First, sit in your chair in a comfortable position with your feet flat on the floor and your hands resting on your knees.

2. Inhale and extend your arms overhead and bring your palms together in a prayer position.

3. Exhale as you bring your hands down to your heart center.

4. Inhale and reach your arms overhead again, stretching your spine.

5. Exhale and hinge forward at your hips and bring your chest toward your thighs.

6. Inhale and lengthen your spine and lift your chest slightly.

7. Exhale and fold forward again and bring your hands to the floor or reaching for your shins.

8. Inhale as you slowly roll back up to a seated position and bring your arms overhead.

9. Repeat the Seated Sun Salutation for 5-10 rounds, coordinating your breath with each movement.

PRECAUTION

Flow through the sequence with ease and avoid rapid motions. If you have joint issues, practice the salutation at a comfortable pace.

CHAIR WARRIOR I VIRABHADRASANA I

In a seated position, extend one leg forward and bend the other, creating a warriorlike stance. Lift your arms overhead, stretching them toward the sky. This pose enhances leg strength and encourages a sense of grounded strength. Switch legs and repeat.

Repetitions: 1 minute

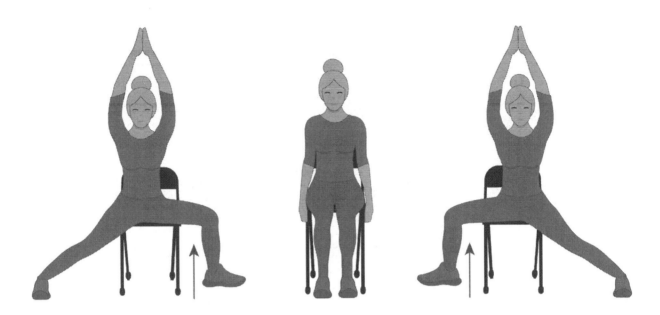

MUSCLES TARGETED

- Quadriceps
- Hip flexors
- Deltoids (shoulders).
- Legs
- Shoulders

INSTRUCTIONS

1. Comfortably sit in your chair with your feet flat on the floor and your spine straight.

2. Extend your right leg straight behind you, keeping the toes on the floor.

3. Bend your left knee and bring it directly over your left ankle.

4. Inhale and raise your arms overhead and bring your palms together.

5. Keep your gaze forward and lift your chest, opening your heart.

6. Hold the Chair Warrior I pose for 20-30 seconds.

7. Exhale and lower your arms and right leg.

8. Repeat on the other side, extending your left leg back and bending your right knee.

9. Inhale slowly as you raise your arms overhead, holding the pose for 20-30 seconds.

10. Release and return to the seated position.

PRECAUTION

Extend arms and lift gently and avoid straining. If you have shoulder or hip concerns, modify the pose and ensure a stable, comfortable stance.

The Only Chair Yoga for Seniors Over 60 Guide You Need

SEATED RUNNING IN PLACE

Seated Running in Place is a dynamic exercise that offers an invigorating cardiovascular workout while being accessible to a wide range of individuals. Tailored for those seeking a seated alternative to traditional running, this activity is particularly beneficial for individuals with mobility challenges or those looking to add variety to their seated exercise routine.

Repetitions: 6 minutes

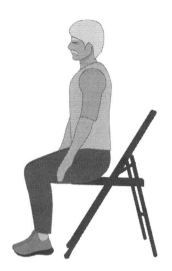 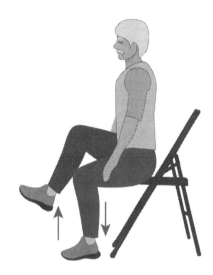

MUSCLES TARGETED

- Quadriceps
- Hamstrings
- Calf muscles
- Cardiovascular system

INSTRUCTIONS

1. Sit in your chair comfortably with your back straight and shoulders relaxed.

2. Place your feet flat on the floor, hip-width apart.

3. Lift your right knee toward your chest and bring it as close as comfortable.

4. As you lower your right foot back to the floor, simultaneously lift your left knee in a running motion.

5. Continue this alternating running motion, lift and lower one knee at a time.

6. Try to match the pace of your movement with the breath while inhaling as you lift and exhaling as you lower.

7. Aim for a brisk but controlled pace that elevates your heart rate without causing discomfort.

8. Feel free to use your arms to mimic a natural running motion, engaging your upper body.

PRECAUTION

Engage in this exercise with caution, especially if you have pre-existing knee or hip issues. adjust the pace to a level that feels challenging yet comfortable, avoiding overexertion.

SEATED CROSS-LEGGED MOUNTAIN CLIMBERS

Seated Cross-Legged Mountain Climbers present an engaging and effective seated exercise suitable for individuals seeking to enhance lower body strength and promote circulation. This variation introduces a cross-legged position, adding a unique twist to the traditional mountain climber movement. Tailored for seniors, this exercise provides a low-impact option to target hip flexors, quadriceps and core muscles.

Repetitions: 45 seconds

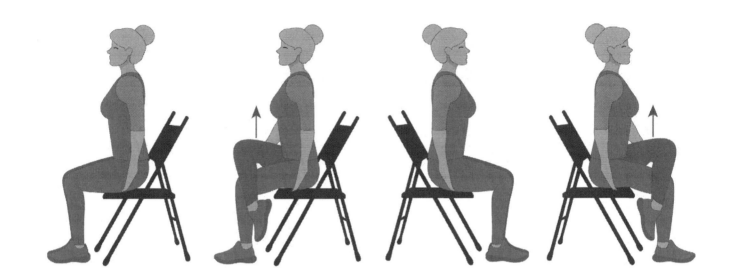

MUSCLES TARGETED

- Hip flexors
- Quadriceps
- Core muscles

INSTRUCTIONS

1. Comfortably sit in your chair with your back straight and shoulders relaxed.
2. Place your feet flat on the floor, hip-width apart.
3. Cross your right leg over your left leg, creating a comfortable cross-legged position.
4. Lift your right knee toward your chest while keeping your foot on the ground.
5. Extend your right leg back to the initial position.
6. Repeat the motion, lift and extend the left knee toward your chest.
7. Continue to switch between the right and left legs, creating a cross-legged mountain climber motion.
8. Coordinate the movement with your breath, inhaling as you lift and exhaling as you extend.

PRECAUTION

Do the seated cross-legged mountain climbers with gentle and controlled movements.

SEATED JAW RELAXATION

Relax your jaw by opening and closing your mouth gently. This exercise helps alleviate jaw tension, especially if you tend to clench your teeth. Take a few moments to breathe deeply and let go of any tension in your jaw.

Repetitions: 60 seconds

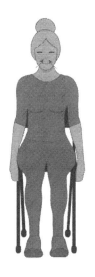 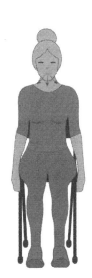

MUSCLES TARGETED

- Jaw muscles
- Facial muscles

INSTRUCTIONS

1. First, sit in your chair in a comfortable position with your back straight and feet flat on the floor.

2. Take a moment to relax your shoulders and release any tension in your neck.

3. Inhale deeply through your nose and as you exhale, allow your jaw to gently drop open.

4. Let your mouth remain slightly open as you inhale and exhale naturally.

5. Close your eyes and focus on softening the muscles in your jaw and face.

6. Hold the relaxed jaw position for 30 seconds, breathing deeply.

7. Gradually close your mouth and bring your awareness back to your surroundings.

8. Perform this exercise as needed to alleviate jaw tension and promote relaxation.

PRECAUTION

Relax the jaw gently and avoid clenching or forcing the jaw open too wide.

SEATED TOE POINT AND FLEX

Seated Toe Point and Flex is a gentle seated exercise designed to promote ankle flexibility and improve circulation, providing a beneficial routine for seniors to maintain lower body mobility.

Repetitions: 8 times per foot

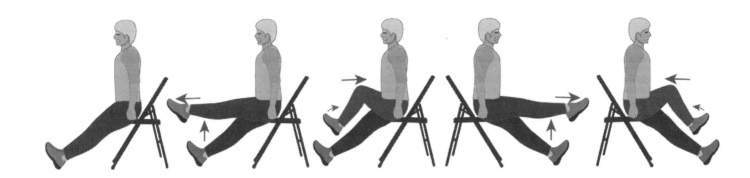

MUSCLES TARGETED

- Ankle flexors and extensors
- Calf muscles

INSTRUCTIONS

1. Comfortably, sit in your chair with your back straight and shoulders relaxed.

2. Keep your feet flat on the floor, maintaining hip-width apart.

3. Lift your right foot off the floor, extending your leg straight.

4. Point your toes forward, stretching the top of your foot, and hold for a moment.

5. Flex your foot back, pulling your toes towards your shin, feeling a stretch in your calf.

6. Return your right foot to the floor and repeat the point and flex movement with your left foot.

7. Continue this alternating point and flex motion, focusing on ankle mobility.

8. Coordinate the movement with your breath, exhaling during the flex and inhaling during the point.

PRECAUTION

Carry out this seated toe point and flex exercise with controlled movements, avoiding any sudden or forceful actions. If you experience discomfort, reduce the range of motion or discontinue the exercise.

The Only Chair Yoga for Seniors Over 60 Guide You Need

SEATED CALF RAISES

Lift your heels off the ground while seated, engaging your calf muscles. This exercise helps improve calf strength and circulation. Lift and lower your heels in a controlled manner and breathe steadily throughout the movement.

Repetitions: 3 sets of 12 raises per calf

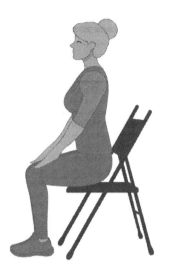 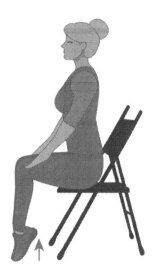 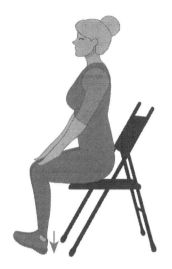

MUSCLES TARGETED

• Calves

INSTRUCTIONS

1. Sit in your chair, in a comfortable position, with your back straight and feet flat on the floor.

2. Put your hands on your thighs for support.

3. Lift your heels off the floor, rising onto the balls of your feet.

4. Hold the raised position for a moment, feeling the contraction in your calf muscles.

5. Lower your heels back down to the floor.

6. Repeat this movement and maintain a controlled pace.

7. Focus on engaging your calf muscles during the upward movement.

8. This exercise helps strengthen the calf muscles and improves ankle mobility.

PRECAUTION

Raise the heels slowly and avoid rapid movements to protect the calf muscles.

LEG PRESS

Seated Leg Press with an extra light resistance band is a beneficial exercise designed to increase muscle strength in the legs and ankles. Sit in a chair with your back straight, holding each end of the resistance band in each hand. Bend one knee towards your chest, raising your foot and place it in the middle of the band. Straighten your knee by kicking forward to stretch against the band, then bend your knee again to return to the starting position. Repeat this process ten times for each leg.

Repetitions: 10 times per leg

Resistance band: Extra Light

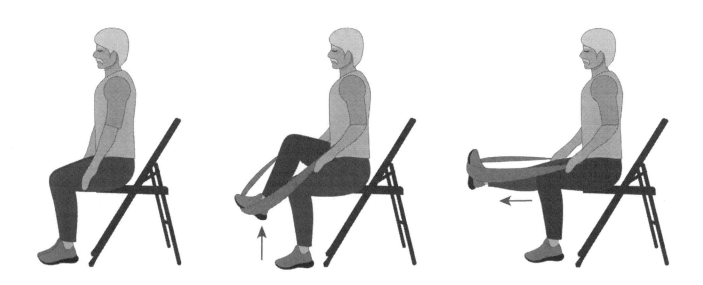

MUSCLES TARGETED

- Quadriceps
- Ankles

INSTRUCTIONS

1. Comfortably, sit in your chair with an upright posture and keep your back straight.

2. Hold each end of the resistance band in each hand, with the band placed under one foot.

3. Bend one knee towards your chest, raise your foot and place it in the middle of the band.

4. Straighten your knee by kicking forward and stretching against the resistance band.

5. Bend your knee again while returning to the starting position.

PRECAUTION

Carry out the leg press with a smooth and controlled motion, avoiding sudden or forceful movements. If you experience discomfort, adjust the resistance band tension or range of motion accordingly.

The Only Chair Yoga for Seniors Over 60 Guide You Need

SEATED HULA HOOP MOTION

Imagine you're gently rotating a hula hoop around your waist while seated. This exercise encourages a subtle twisting motion, promoting flexibility in your spine and engaging your core muscles. Move in a circular pattern, enjoying the fluidity of the movement.

Repetitions: 2 minutes

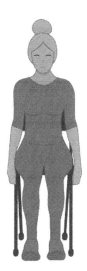 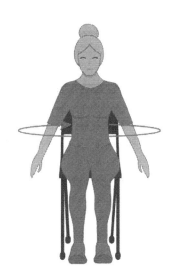 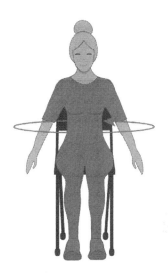

MUSCLES TARGETED

- Core muscles
- Abdominal muscles

INSTRUCTIONS

1. Sit in your chair, in a comfortable position, with your back straight and feet flat on the floor.

2. Imagine holding a hula hoop in your hands, palms facing each other.

3. Start rotating your upper body as if you are moving a hula hoop in a circular motion.

4. Coordinate the movement with your torso, engaging your core muscles.

5. Continue the circular motion for 2 minutes, alternating between clockwise and counter-clockwise directions.

6. Keep your pace smooth and deliberate during the exercise.

PRECAUTION

Move hips gently as if using a hula hoop and avoid sharp or exaggerated motions.

28-DAY INTERMEDIATE CHAIR YOGA CHALLENGE

WEEK 01

Days	Warm-Up	Heart Health	Bad posture	Weight-loss	Joint Mobility
Monday	Seated Side Leg Lifts **p.44**	Seated Side Leg Raises **p.49**	Seated Leg Cross Toe Touches **p.55**	Seated Cross-legged Arm Twist **p.59**	Seated Calf Raises **p.67**
Tuesday	Chair Tap Dance **p.45**	Seated Chest Expansion **p.50**	Seated Side Bend **p.56**	Seated Warrior II **p.60**	Leg Press **p.68**
Wednesday	Seated Rowing **p.46**	Seated Quadriceps Stretch **p.51**	Seated Cactus Arms **p.57**	Seated Sun Salutation (Surya Namaskar) **p.61**	Seated Hula Hoop Motion **p.69**
Thursday	Seated Bicycle Crunches **p.47**	Seated Prayer Twist **p.52**	Seated Wall Angels **p.58**	Chair Warrior I Virabhadrasana I **p.62**	Seated Jaw Relaxation **p.65**
Friday	Seated Side Leg Cross **p.48**	Seated Lateral Arm Raises **p.53**	Seated Balance Pose with Arm Reach **p.54**	Seated Running in Place **p.63**	Seated Toe Point and Flex **p.66**
Saturday	Seated Side Leg Lifts **p.44**	Seated Side Leg Raises **p.49**	Seated Leg Cross Toe Touches **p.55**	Seated Cross-Legged Mountain Climbers **p.64**	Seated Calf Raises **p.67**
Sunday	Chair Tap Dance **p.45**	Seated Chest Expansion **p.50**	Seated Side Bend **p.56**	Seated Cross-Legged Mountain Climbers **p.64**	Leg Press **p.68**

The Only Chair Yoga for Seniors Over 60 Guide You Need

WEEK 02

Days	Warm-Up	Heart Health	Bad posture	Weight-loss	Joint Mobility
Monday	Seated Bicycle Crunches **p.47**	Seated Chest Expansion **p.50**	Seated Balance Pose with Arm Reach **p.54**	Seated Warrior II **p.60**	Seated Jaw Relaxation **p.65**
Tuesday	Seated Side Leg Cross **p.48**	Seated Quadriceps Stretch **p.51**	Seated Leg Cross Toe Touches **p.55**	Seated Sun Salutation (Surya Namaskar) **p.61**	Seated Toe Point and Flex **p.66**
Wednesday	Chair Tap Dance **p.45**	Seated Prayer Twist **p.52**	Seated Side Bend **p.56**	Chair Warrior I Virabhadrasana I **p.62**	Seated Calf Raises **p.67**
Thursday	Seated Rowing **p.46**	Seated Lateral Arm Raises **p.53**	Seated Cactus Arms **p.57**	Seated Cross-legged Arm Twist **p.59**	Leg Press **p.68**
Friday	Seated Side Leg Lifts **p.44**	Seated Side Leg Raises **p.49**	Seated Wall Angels **p.58**	Seated Running in Place **p.63**	Seated Hula Hoop Motion **p.69**
Saturday	Seated Bicycle Crunches **p.47**	Seated Chest Expansion **p.50**	Seated Balance Pose with Arm Reach **p.54**	Seated Cross-Legged Mountain Climbers **p.64**	Seated Jaw Relaxation **p.65**
Sunday	Seated Side Leg Cross **p.48**	Seated Quadriceps Stretch **p.51**	Seated Leg Cross Toe Touches **p.55**	Seated Warrior II **p.60**	Seated Toe Point and Flex **p.66**

WEEK 03

Days	Warm-Up	Heart Health	Bad posture	Weight-loss	Joint Mobility
Monday	Seated Side Leg Lifts **p.44**	Seated Side Leg Raises **p.49**	Seated Leg Cross Toe Touches **p.55**	Seated Cross-legged Arm Twist **p.59**	Seated Calf Raises **p.67**
Tuesday	Chair Tap Dance **p.45**	Seated Chest Expansion **p.50**	Seated Side Bend **p.56**	Seated Warrior II **p.60**	Leg Press **p.68**
Wednes-day	Seated Rowing **p.46**	Seated Quadri-ceps Stretch **p.51**	Seated Cactus Arms **p.57**	Seated Sun Sal-utation (Surya Namaskar) **p.61**	Seated Hula Hoop Motion **p.69**
Thursday	Seated Bicycle Crunches **p.47**	Seated Prayer Twist **p.52**	Seated Wall Angels **p.58**	Chair Warrior I Virabhadrasa-na I **p.62**	Seated Jaw Re-laxation **p.65**
Friday	Seated Side Leg Cross **p.48**	Seated Lateral Arm Raises **p.53**	Seated Balance Pose with Arm Reach **p.54**	Seated Running in Place **p.63**	Seated Toe Point and Flex **p.66**
Saturday	Seated Side Leg Lifts **p.44**	Seated Side Leg Raises **p.49**	Seated Leg Cross Toe Touches **p.55**	Seated Cross-Legged Moun-tain Climbers **p.64**	Seated Calf Raises **p.67**
Sunday	Chair Tap Dance **p.45**	Seated Chest Expansion **p.50**	Seated Side Bend **p.56**	Seated Sun Sal-utation (Surya Namaskar) **p.61**	Leg Press **p.68**

WEEK 04

Days	Warm-Up	Heart Health	Bad posture	Weight-loss	Joint Mobility
Monday	Seated Bicycle Crunches **p.47**	Seated Prayer Twist **p.52**	Seated Balance Pose with Arm Reach **p.54**	Seated Warrior II **p.60**	Seated Jaw Relaxation **p.65**
Tuesday	Seated Side Leg Cross **p.48**	Seated Quadriceps Stretch **p.51**	Seated Leg Cross Toe Touches **p.55**	Seated Sun Salutation (Surya Namaskar) **p.61**	Seated Toe Point and Flex **p.66**
Wednesday	Chair Tap Dance **p.45**	Seated Prayer Twist **p.52**	Seated Side Bend **p.56**	Chair Warrior I Virabhadrasana I **p.62**	Seated Calf Raises **p.67**
Thursday	Seated Rowing **p.46**	Seated Lateral Arm Raises **p.53**	Seated Cactus Arms **p.57**	Seated Running in Place **p.63**	Leg Press **p.68**
Friday	Chair Tap Dance **p.45**	Seated Side Leg Raises **p.49**	Seated Wall Angels **p.58**	Seated Cross-Legged Mountain Climbers **p.64**	Seated Hula Hoop Motion **p.69**
Saturday	Seated Bicycle Crunches **p.47**	Seated Chest Expansion **p.50**	Seated Balance Pose with Arm Reach **p.54**	Seated Cross-legged Arm Twist **p.59**	Seatjawed Jaw Relaxation **p.65**
Sunday	Seated Side Leg Cross **p.48**	Seated Quadriceps Stretch **p.51**	Seated Leg Cross Toe Touches **p.55**	Seated Warrior II **p.60**	Seated Toe Point and Flex **p.66**

CHAPTER 5:
CHALLENGE YOURSELF WITH ADVANCED POSES

POSES TO WARM-UP

HALF LIFT (ARDHA UTTANASANA)

Seated Half Lift or Ardha Uttanasana, is a gentle yoga pose that provides a subtle yet effective stretch for the muscles in your lower back and hamstrings. This seated variation is perfect for seniors and allows you to experience the benefits of a half lift while sitting comfortably in a chair. The pose is designed to promote flexibility in the spine and hamstrings, offering relief from stiffness and tension.

Repetitions: 10 times

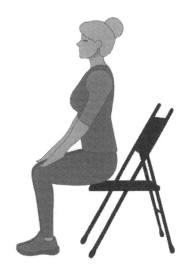 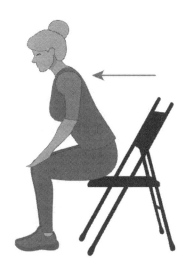

MUSCLES TARGETED

- Erector spinae
- Hamstrings
- Glutes

INSTRUCTIONS

1. Sit on the edge of a chair with your feet flat on the floor and hip-width apart.
2. Inhale and lengthen your spine, sitting tall.
3. Put your hands on your thighs for support.
4. Exhale and hinge at your hips, leaning forward slightly.

5. Lift your chest and extend your torso forward, creating a straight line from your tailbone to the crown of your head.
6. Hold the stretch for 15-30 seconds, feeling a gentle pull along your lower back and hamstrings.
7. Inhale as you slowly return to an upright position.

PRECAUTION

Keep a flat back; don't overextend or strain your spine.

The Only Chair Yoga for Seniors Over 60 Guide You Need

COBRA POSE (BHUJANGASANA)

Seated Cobra Pose or Bhujangasana, is a wonderful yoga-inspired exercise that promotes spinal flexibility and strengthens the muscles in your back and shoulders. This modified cobra pose can be comfortably performed while sitting in a chair, making it accessible for seniors. By incorporating Seated Cobra, you engage the muscles along your spine, helping to alleviate stiffness and improve posture.

Repetitions: 15 times

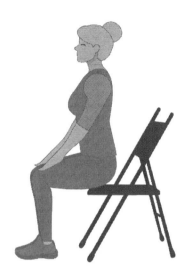 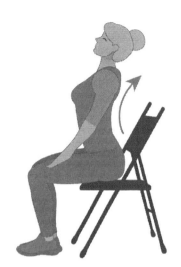

MUSCLES TARGETED

- Erector spinae
- Rectus abdominis
- Muscles of the lower back

INSTRUCTIONS

1. Sit on the edge of a chair with your feet flat on the floor and your hands resting on your thighs.

2. Inhale deeply and engage your core muscles.

3. Exhale as you gently arch your back and lift your chest toward the ceiling.

4. Keep your shoulders down and away from your ears.

5. Allow your head to tilt backward slightly, gazing upward.

6. Hold the pose for 10-15 seconds, feeling a gentle stretch along your spine.

7. Inhale slowly as you return to an upright seated position.

PRECAUTION

Lift with your back muscles, not just your hands and avoid straining your lower back.

KUNDALINI CIRCLES (SEATED TORSO CIRCLES)

Seated Kundalini Circles, also known as Seated Torso Circles, is a dynamic and invigorating exercise designed to enhance flexibility and vitality, particularly in the torso and spine. This exercise draws inspiration from Kundalini yoga practices, promoting a sense of flow and energy within the body.

Repetitions: 8 times in each direction

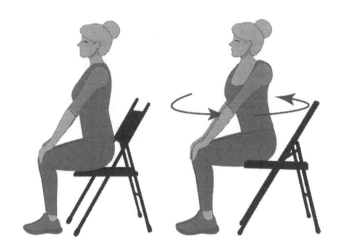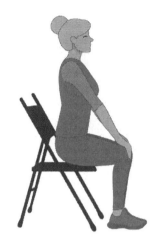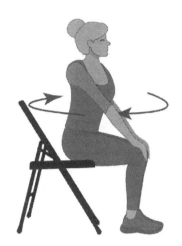

MUSCLES TARGETED

- Core muscles
- Spinal muscles
- Obliques

INSTRUCTIONS

1. Comfortably, sit in your chair with a tall spine and relaxed shoulders.

2. Keep your feet flat on the floor, maintaining hip-width apart.

3. Place your hands on your knees or thighs for support.

4. Initiate the movement by gently circling your torso to the right, creating a circular motion.

5. Continue the circular motion, making a full rotation to the right.

6. Reverse the direction and circle your torso to the left, completing a full rotation in that direction.

7. Engage your core muscles throughout the exercise to support your spine.

PRECAUTION

Carry out these seated torso circles with controlled movements, avoiding any sudden or forceful actions. If you experience discomfort, reduce the size of the circles or discontinue the exercise.

The Only Chair Yoga for Seniors Over 60 Guide You Need

SEATED SHOULDER STRETCH

Seated Shoulder Stretch is a gentle and effective exercise designed to relieve tension and enhance flexibility in the shoulder muscles. This seated stretch is suitable for individuals of all fitness levels and can be particularly beneficial for those who spend long hours at a desk or engaged in activities that may cause shoulder stiffness.

Repetitions: 2-3 sets of 15 seconds per side

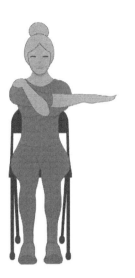 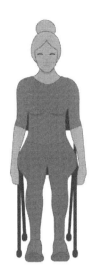 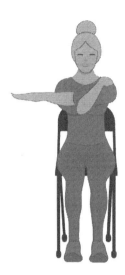

MUSCLES TARGETED

- Shoulders
- Upper back
- Neck muscles

INSTRUCTIONS

1. Sit in your chair, in a comfortable position, with your back straight and shoulders relaxed.
2. Place your feet flat on the floor, hip-width apart.
3. Reach your right arm across your chest, keeping it straight.
4. Use your left hand to gently press against the outer part of your right upper arm, near the shoulder.

5. Feel the stretch in your right shoulder and hold for 15 seconds, avoiding any pain.
6. Release the stretch and repeat the same motion on the left side while reaching your left arm across and using your right hand to press gently.
7. Alternate between right and left stretches for a total of three sets.

PRECAUTION

Practice the shoulder stretches with gentle and controlled movements.

Avoid bouncing or jerky motions during the stretch to prevent injury.

SEATED HEEL SLIDES

Seated Heel Slides offer a seated exercise option designed to improve lower body flexibility and engage the muscles in the thighs and lower legs. This exercise is suitable for individuals of various fitness levels and can be particularly helpful for those looking to enhance mobility in the hip and knee joints.

Repetitions: 2 sets of 12 slides on each leg

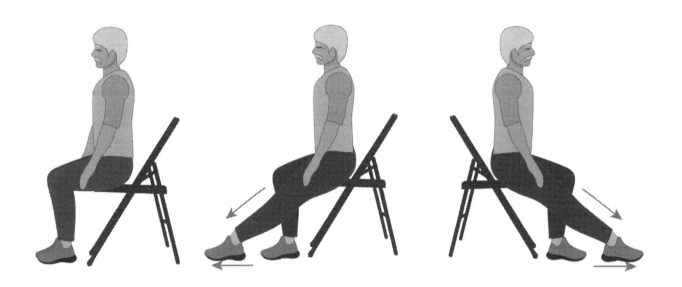

MUSCLES TARGETED

- Hip flexors
- Quadriceps
- Hamstrings

INSTRUCTIONS

1. Comfortably sit in your chair with your back straight and shoulders relaxed.

2. Place your feet flat on the floor and maintain a hip-width distance between them.

3. Slide your right heel forward along the floor, straightening your right knee.

4. Return your right foot to the starting position and keep your motion controlled.

5. Repeat the sliding motion with your left heel, straightening your left knee.

6. Continue to switch between right and left heel slides for a set of 12 on each leg.

7. Coordinate the slides with your breath, exhaling as you extend your leg and inhaling as you return to the starting position.

PRECAUTION

Do the heel slides with controlled movements to avoid any strain or injury.

If you have any knee issues, limit the range of motion to a point that is comfortable for you.

Maintain proper posture throughout the exercise to maximize its effectiveness.

SEATED STAR POSE

Seated Star Pose is a rejuvenating and accessible exercise designed for seniors to enhance lower body strength and stimulate circulation. This seated posture engages various muscle groups, focusing on the hip flexors, quadriceps and core muscles.

Repetitions: 90 seconds

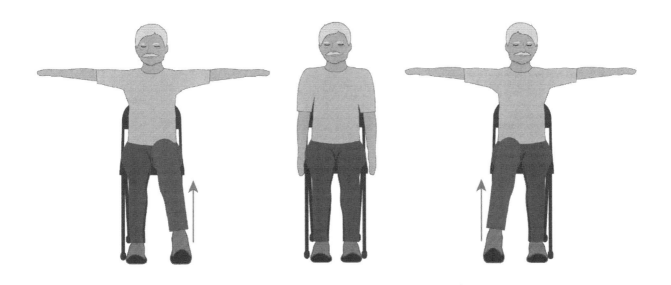

MUSCLES TARGETED

- Hip flexors
- Quadriceps
- Core muscles

INSTRUCTIONS

1. Sit in your chair, in a comfortable position, with your back straight and shoulders relaxed.

2. Place your feet flat on the floor and maintain a hip-width distance between them.

3. Extend your arms out to the sides, creating a starlike shape with your body.

4. Inhale slowly as you lift your right knee towards your chest, keeping your foot on the ground.

5. Exhale and gently lower your right foot back to the floor.

6. Repeat the motion with your left knee and lift it towards your chest.

7. Continue this alternating motion, creating a rhythmic pattern resembling a seated star.

PRECAUTION

Lift your knees gently to avoid sudden or forceful movements. If you experience discomfort or pain, modify the range of motion or consult with a healthcare professional. Adjust the pace according to your comfort level and individual capabilities.

SEATED EAGLE ARMS

Seated Eagle Arms offers a soothing and beneficial exercise designed for seniors to enhance upper body flexibility and promote relaxation. This seated pose primarily targets the muscles in the arms, shoulders and upper back.

Repetitions: 60 seconds

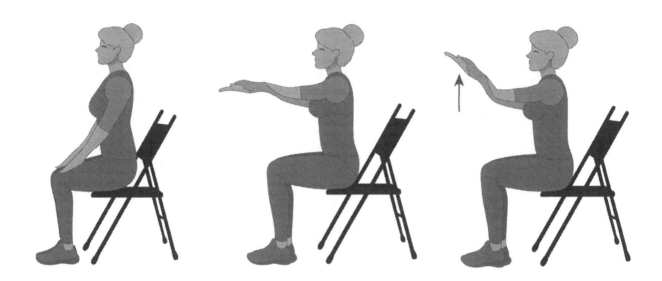

MUSCLES TARGETED

- Arms
- Shoulders
- Upper back

INSTRUCTIONS

1. First, sit in your chair in a comfortable position with your back straight and shoulders relaxed.

2. Place your feet flat on the floor and maintain a hip-width distance between them.

3. Inhale deeply as you raise your arms to shoulder height, extending them straight in front of you.

4. Exhale and cross your right arm over the left and bring the palms of your hands together.

5. If possible, entwine your forearms and press your palms together, creating an "eagle arm" position.

6. Lift your elbows slightly while maintaining a gentle stretch across the upper back and shoulders.

7. Hold this position for a few breaths, feeling the stretch in your upper arms and shoulders.

8. Inhale slowly as you release the arms, extending them straight out in front of you again.

9. Repeat the process, crossing the left arm over the right this time.

PRECAUTION

Practice the movement with a gentle and controlled pace to avoid strain. If you experience discomfort, modify the arm positions or reduce the range of motion. Be mindful of any shoulder or arm issues, adjusting the exercise accordingly.

The Only Chair Yoga for Seniors Over 60 Guide You Need

SEATED WARRIOR III

Seated Warrior III is a rejuvenating exercise designed to enhance balance, strengthen the lower body and engage core muscles. It offers a modified version of the traditional Warrior III pose, tailored for individuals who prefer or require a seated position.

Repetitions: 90 seconds

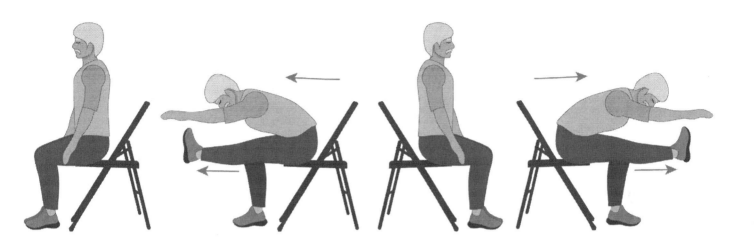

MUSCLES TARGETED

- Hip flexors
- Quadriceps
- Core muscles

INSTRUCTIONS

1. Comfortably sit in your chair with your back straight and shoulders relaxed.

2. Place your feet flat on the floor and maintain a hip-width distance between them.

3. Engage your core muscles for stability.

4. Extend your right leg straight out in front of you, hovering above the floor.

5. Point your toes and keep the leg in line with your hip and form a straight line from your head to your extended foot.

6. Simultaneously, lean forward slightly and bring your torso closer to your thigh while keeping your back straight.

7. Extend your arms forward or put your hands on the sides of the chair for support.

8. Hold this position for a few breaths, feeling the engagement in your hip, thigh and core.

9. Return your right foot to the floor and repeat the movement on the left side.

10. Alternate between the right and left legs, creating a flowing and controlled motion.

PRECAUTION

Practice the exercise at a pace that feels comfortable and controlled.

Avoid sudden or forceful movements, especially when extending your legs.

If you experience discomfort, adjust the range of motion or modify the pose as needed.

SEATED FIGURE FOUR STRETCH

Seated Figure Four Stretch is a gentle yet effective exercise aimed at improving hip flexibility and providing relief to the muscles around the hip and lower back. This stretch is particularly beneficial for individuals who may experience tightness in the hips.

Repetitions: Hold each stretch for 15-30 seconds, repeat 5 times per side

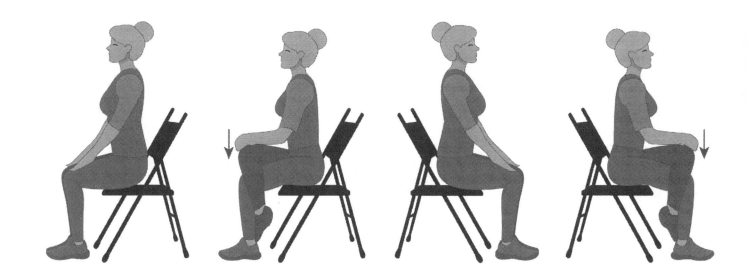

MUSCLES TARGETED

- Hip flexors
- Quadriceps
- Core muscles

INSTRUCTIONS

1. Sit in your chair, in a comfortable position, with your back straight and shoulders relaxed.

2. Place your feet flat on the floor and maintain a hip-width distance between them.

3. Lift your right foot off the floor and cross it over your left thigh and form a "Figure Four" shape with your legs.

4. Flex your right foot to protect your knee and enhance the stretch.

5. Gently press on your right knee with your hand to encourage a deeper stretch. Keep your back straight during the stretch.

6. You should feel a gentle stretch in the outer hip of the crossed leg.

7. Hold the stretch for 15-30 seconds, focusing on your breath.

8. Release the stretch and repeat on the other side, crossing your left foot over your right thigh.

PRECAUTION

Do the stretch in a controlled and gradual manner.

Avoid sudden or forceful movements and allow the muscles to relax into the stretch.

The Only Chair Yoga for Seniors Over 60 Guide You Need

SEATED MOUNTAIN CLIMBERS

Seated Mountain Climbers offer a seated adaptation of the classic exercise, providing a dynamic way to engage the core and elevate the heart rate. This modified version is well-suited for individuals looking to enhance their cardiovascular fitness and strengthen core muscles while remaining seated.

Repetitions: 90 seconds

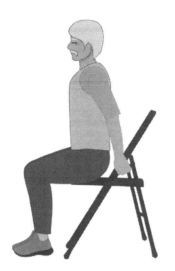 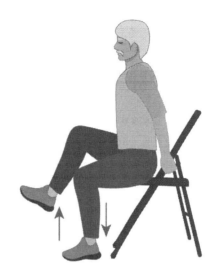

MUSCLES TARGETED

- Hip flexors
- Quadriceps
- Core muscles

INSTRUCTIONS

1. Sit in your chair, in a comfortable position, with your back straight and shoulders relaxed.

2. Place your feet flat on the floor and maintain a hip-width apart stance.

3. Rest your hands on the sides of the chair for stability.

4. Lift your right knee toward your chest, engaging your core muscles.

5. Lower your right foot back to the floor and swiftly lift your left knee toward your chest.

6. Alternate the movement, resembling a marching motion with a brisk but controlled pace.

7. Coordinate the knee lifts with your breath, inhaling as you lift and exhaling as you lower.

8. Aim for a smooth, rhythmic sequence while keeping the upper body stable.

PRECAUTION

Lift your knees gently and avoid sudden or forceful movements.

Maintain proper posture with your back straight throughout the exercise.

If you experience discomfort or pain, adjust the pace or range of motion.

SEATED RIBCAGE SIDE STRETCH

Seated Ribcage Side Stretch is a soothing exercise designed to enhance flexibility and mobility in the upper body, specifically targeting the ribcage and side muscles. This seated stretch is well-suited for seniors, offering a gentle way to promote better posture and alleviate tension.

Repetitions: 10 times per side

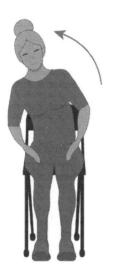 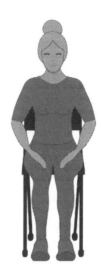 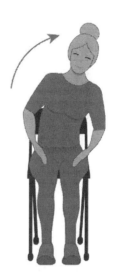

MUSCLES TARGETED

- Ribcage muscles
- Side muscles (obliques)
- Upper back muscles

INSTRUCTIONS

1. Comfortably sit in your chair with your back straight and shoulders relaxed.

2. Place your feet flat on the floor and maintain hip-width apart.

3. Inhale deeply and elongate your spine.

4. As you exhale, gently lean your upper body to the right, creating a lateral stretch along your left side.

5. Hold the stretch for a few breaths, feeling the gentle elongation along the left side of your ribcage.

6. Inhale slowly as you return to the upright position.

7. Repeat the stretch, this time leaning to the left and feeling the stretch along your right side.

8. Coordinate the stretch with your breath, inhaling during the upright position and exhaling during the stretch.

9. Aim for a smooth and controlled motion that feels comfortable for your flexibility.

PRECAUTION

Carry out the stretch with gentle and gradual movements, avoiding any sudden or forceful motions.

If you have any existing back issues or injuries, modify the stretch to ensure comfort.

CHEST PRESS

Seated Chest Press is a chest strengthening exercise that mirrors the traditional bench press, designed to fortify chest muscles while allowing you to stay comfortably seated. Secure a resistance band around the back of your chair, approximately at chest level. Grasp both ends of the band with your hands, starting with your elbows bent and hands towards your chest.

Repetitions: 10 times

Resistance band: Extra Light

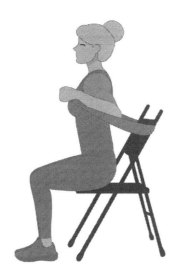 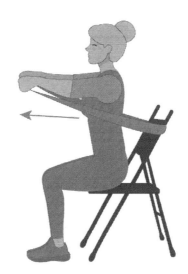

MUSCLES TARGETED

- Pectoral muscles (chest)
- Anterior deltoids (front shoulders)

INSTRUCTIONS

1. Comfortably, sit in your chair with an upright posture and secure a resistance band around the back of the chair at chest level.

2. Hold both ends of the band with your hands and start with your elbows bent and hands close to your chest.

3. Push your hands forward away from your chest and feel the resistance in your chest muscles.

4. Bend your elbows to bring your hands back towards your chest and maintain control throughout the movement.

PRECAUTION

Pay attention to your form and avoid using excessive force. If you experience any discomfort, modify the tension or range of motion.

SEATED LATERAL BAND

Seated Lateral Band is a beneficial exercise that targets both upper and lower leg muscles, enhancing strength and flexibility. Start by bringing both legs and knees together in front of you while seated. Wrap a resistance band around your thighs, just above the knees, adjusting the tension to your preference and securing it with a knot.

Repetitions: 10 times (alternating legs)

Resistance band: Extra Light

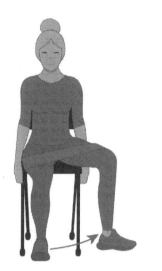 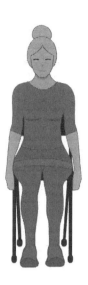 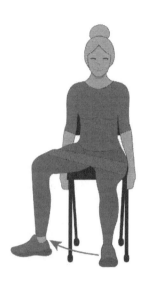

MUSCLES TARGETED

- Inner and outer thigh muscles
- Quadriceps

INSTRUCTIONS

1. Comfortably, sit in your chair with an upright posture then bring both legs and knees together in front of you.

2. Wrap a resistance band around your thighs, just above the knees and tighten it to your desired level.

3. Secure the band with a knot to keep it in place during the exercise.

4. Move one leg to the side and away from your body as far as possible and engage your thigh muscles.

5. Return that leg to the starting position in front of you.

6. Repeat the lateral leg movement with the other leg.

PRECAUTION

Carry out the lateral leg movements with controlled motions to avoid strain. If you experience discomfort, adjust the resistance band tension accordingly.

SEATED CHIN TUCKS

Seated Chin Tucks are a simple yet effective exercise designed to improve neck mobility and alleviate tension in the cervical spine. This seated variation is particularly beneficial for seniors who may experience stiffness in the neck due to prolonged periods of sitting or poor posture. By incorporating Seated Chin Tucks into your routine, you target the muscles in the neck and upper back, promoting better alignment and reducing discomfort.

Repetitions: 20 times

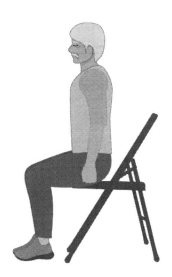 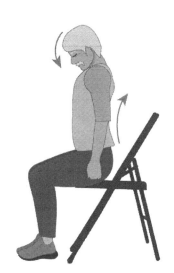

MUSCLES TARGETED

- Sternocleidomastoid
- Neck flexors
- Upper back

INSTRUCTIONS

1. First, sit in your chair in a comfortable position with your back straight and your feet flat on the floor.

2. Deeply inhale the air and lengthen your spine.

3. Exhale as you gently lower your chin toward your chest, keeping your movements slow and controlled.

4. Hold the tucked position for 5-10 seconds, feeling a stretch along the back of your neck.

5. Inhale again as you lift your head back to the neutral position.

6. Pay attention to keeping your shoulders relaxed and avoiding any discomfort in the neck.

PRECAUTION

Tuck the chin gently and avoid straining the neck. If you have neck concerns, keep the movements small and controlled.

SEATED RHOMBOID SQUEEZE

The Seated Rhomboid Squeeze is a fantastic exercise designed to strengthen the muscles between your shoulder blades, known as the rhomboids. This seated variation is especially beneficial for seniors looking to improve their upper back strength and posture.

Repetitions: 20 times

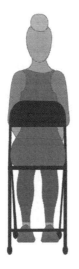 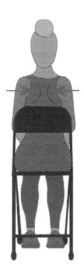

MUSCLES TARGETED

- Rhomboids
- Middle trapezius
- Upper back

INSTRUCTIONS

1. Sit in your chair, in a comfortable position, with your back straight and your feet flat on the floor.

2. Deeply inhale the air and lengthen your spine.

3. Exhale as you gently squeeze your shoulder blades together, as if you're trying to hold a small object between them.

4. Hold the squeezed position for 5-10 seconds, feeling the contraction in your upper back.

5. Inhale again as you release the squeeze and allow your shoulder blades to naturally separate.

6. Repeat the movement for 20 repetitions and maintain a slow and controlled pace.

7. Focus on keeping your neck and shoulders relaxed throughout the exercise.

PRECAUTION

Squeeze the shoulder blades gently and avoid tensing. If you have back problems, carry out the movement with a focus on stability.

The Only Chair Yoga for Seniors Over 60 Guide You Need

SEATED TORSO TWIST PUNCHES

Seated Torso Twist Punches add a dynamic twist to your seated workout routine, engaging your core muscles, shoulders and promoting flexibility in the torso. This exercise combines the benefits of torso twisting with the added element of punching, providing a comprehensive upper-body workout for individuals looking to stay active while seated.

Repetitions: 12 times per side

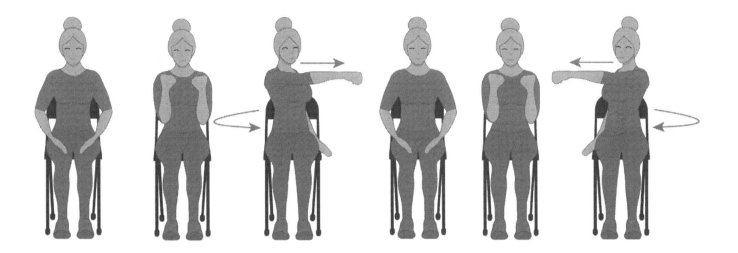

MUSCLES TARGETED

- Abdominals (Rectus Abdominis and Obliques)
- Shoulders
- Back muscles

INSTRUCTIONS

1. Sit in your chair, in a comfortable position, with your back straight and shoulders relaxed.
2. Place your feet flat on the floor, hip-width apart while making sure that you have a stable base.
3. Extend your arms in front of you and form fists with your hands.
4. Twist your torso to the right, engaging your abdominal muscles.

5. Simultaneously, punch your right fist towards the right side.
6. Return your right fist to the center as you untwist your torso.
7. Repeat the sequence on the left side, twist to the left and punch with your left fist.
8. In an alternate movement, switch between right and left torso twists with punches for a total of 12 repetitions per side.

PRECAUTION

Perform torso twists and punches with controlled and deliberate movements to avoid strain.

SEATED LEG CROSS AND REACH

Seated Leg Cross and Reach is a seated exercise that combines leg crossing with a reaching motion, offering a beneficial stretch for the lower body and engaging core muscles. This movement is suitable for individuals looking to enhance flexibility, improve hip mobility and strengthen the abdominal muscles while remaining comfortably seated.

Repetitions: 12 times per leg

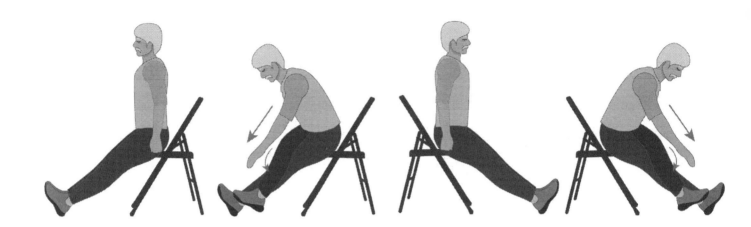

MUSCLES TARGETED

- Hip flexors
- Quadriceps
- Hamstrings
- Abdominals (Rectus Abdominis)

INSTRUCTIONS

1. Sit in your chair, in a comfortable position, with your back straight and shoulders relaxed.

2. Place your feet flat on the floor, hip-width apart while making sure that you have a stable base.

3. Lift your right knee toward your chest, crossing it over your left leg.

4. Simultaneously, reach your right hand towards your left foot, engaging your abdominal muscles.

5. Feel a gentle stretch in your hip flexors and hamstrings as you reach.

6. Return your right foot to the floor and repeat the motion on the left side, lift your left knee and reach towards your right foot.

7. In an alternate movement, switch between leg crosses and reaches for a total of 12 repetitions on each leg.

8. Coordinate the movements with your breath, exhaling as you reach and inhaling during the return to the starting position.

PRECAUTION

Carry out the leg crosses and reaches with controlled movements to avoid any sudden or forceful motions.

The Only Chair Yoga for Seniors Over 60 Guide You Need

SEATED MOUNTAIN POSE WITH ARM REACH

Seated Mountain Pose with Arm Reach is a soothing and beneficial exercise, especially suitable for individuals seeking a seated practice to enhance overall body flexibility and mindfulness. This pose incorporates a gentle stretch and extension of the arms, promoting relaxation and improved posture.

Repetitions: 5 times per side

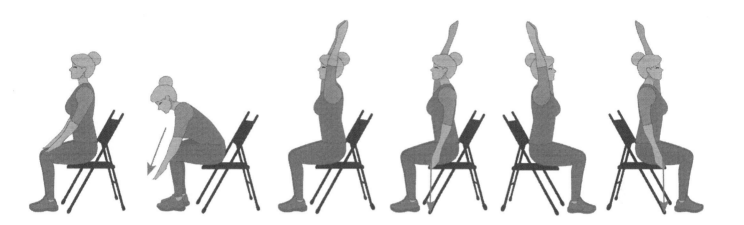

MUSCLES TARGETED

- Spine
- Shoulders
- Arms (Triceps and Biceps)

INSTRUCTIONS

1. First, sit in your chair in a comfortable position with your back straight and shoulders relaxed.

2. Place your feet flat on the floor, hip-width apart and maintain a stable and grounded posture.

3. Extend both arms alongside your body while reaching them towards the floor with palms facing inward.

4. Inhale deeply as you lift both arms overhead and bring your palms to touch.

5. Exhale slowly as you lower your right arm down the side of your body while reaching towards the floor.

6. Maintain the stretch, feeling a gentle elongation along the left side of your torso and arm.

7. Inhale slowly as you return both arms overhead, palms together.

8. Exhale and repeat the stretch on the opposite side, lowering your left arm towards the floor.

9. Continue to switch sides, syncing the movement with your breath.

PRECAUTION

Execute the movements with gentle and deliberate motions, avoiding any abrupt or forceful stretches.

SEATED KNEE LIFTS WITH TWIST

Seated Knee Lifts with Twist is a dynamic and engaging exercise designed to enhance mobility, flexibility and core strength. This seated movement incorporates a twisting motion, adding an extra element to the traditional knee lifts. It's an excellent choice for individuals seeking to improve their abdominal strength and overall seated workout experience.

Repetitions: 10 times per side

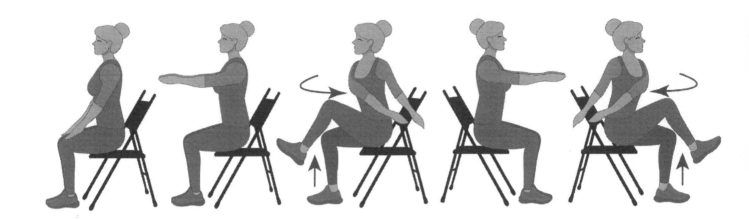

MUSCLES TARGETED

- Abdominals (Rectus Abdominis and Obliques)
- Hip flexors
- Quadriceps

INSTRUCTIONS

1. Sit in your chair, in a comfortable position, with your back straight and shoulders relaxed.

2. Place your feet flat on the floor, hip-width apart while making sure that you have a stable base.

3. Extend your arms straight in front of you, palms facing each other.

4. Lift your right knee toward your chest while simultaneously twisting your torso to the right.

5. Return your right foot to the floor and repeat the motion on the left side, lift your left knee and twist to the left.

6. Continue this alternating motion, lift and twist with each knee lift.

7. Keep your pace controlled and focus on engaging your core muscles during the exercise.

PRECAUTION

Execute the knee lifts and twists with controlled and deliberate movements to avoid strain.

SEATED QUADRICEPS ACTIVATION

Seated Quadriceps Activation is a targeted exercise designed to engage and strengthen the quadriceps muscles while seated in a chair. This focused movement not only enhances lower body strength but also serves as an excellent option for individuals with mobility limitations.

Repetitions: 45 seconds

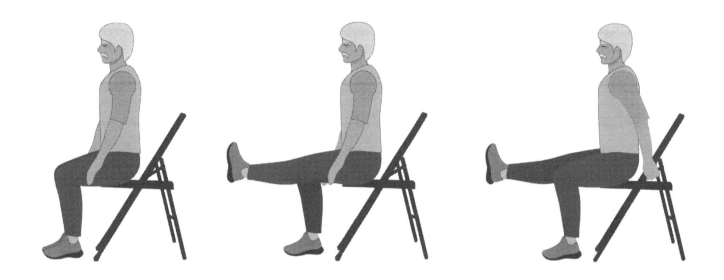

MUSCLES TARGETED

- Quadriceps
- Hip flexors
- Core muscles

INSTRUCTIONS

1. Sit in your chair comfortably with your back straight and shoulders relaxed.
2. Place your feet flat on the floor and keep them hip-width apart for a stable posture.
3. Extend your right leg straight in front of you, contracting the quadriceps muscles.

4. Hold the extended position briefly, focusing on the engagement in your quadriceps.
5. Lower your right leg back to the floor and repeat the motion with your left leg.
6. Continue this alternating leg extension, emphasizing the contraction in the quadriceps.

PRECAUTION

Practice the leg extensions with controlled movements, avoiding any sudden or jerky motions.

SEATED LATERAL ARM RAISES WITH LEG CROSS

This exercise combines the benefits of lateral arm raises with a leg crossing motion, promoting coordination and targeting multiple muscle groups.

Repetitions: 20 times per arm

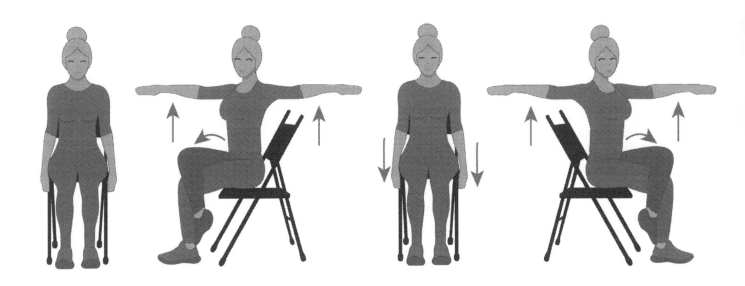

MUSCLES TARGETED

- Deltoids (shoulder muscles)
- Latissimus dorsi (upper back muscles)
- Abdominals
- Hip abductors (outer thigh muscles)

INSTRUCTIONS

1. Sit in your chair, in a comfortable position, with an upright posture and make sure that your back is straight.

2. Place your feet flat on the floor, hip-width apart.

3. Extend your arms straight out to the sides at shoulder height, palms facing down.

4. While maintaining the arm position, lift your right leg and cross it over your left leg.

5. Return your right foot to the floor and repeat the motion, this time lifting your left leg and crossing it over your right leg.

6. Continue to switch the leg cross while performing lateral arm raises.

PRECAUTION

Do the leg cross and arm raises with controlled movements to prevent any sudden or jerky motions, especially if you have joint issues or discomfort.

The Only Chair Yoga for Seniors Over 60 Guide You Need

LEG PRESS

Seated Leg Press with an extra light resistance band is a beneficial exercise designed to increase muscle strength in the legs and ankles. Sit in a chair with your back straight, holding each end of the resistance band in each hand. Bend one knee towards your chest, raising your foot and place it in the middle of the band. Straighten your knee by kicking forward to stretch against the band, then bend your knee again to return to the starting position. Repeat this process ten times for each leg.

Repetitions: 10 times per leg

Resistance band: Extra Light

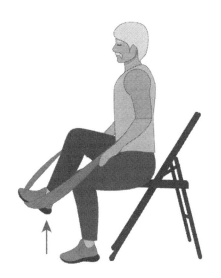 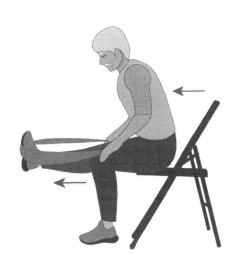

MUSCLES TARGETED

- Quadriceps
- Ankles

INSTRUCTIONS

1. Comfortably, sit in your chair with an upright posture and keep your back is straight.

2. Hold each end of the resistance band in each hand, with the band placed under one foot.

3. Bend one knee towards your chest, raise your foot and place it in the middle of the band.

4. Straighten your knee by kicking forward and stretching against the resistance band.

5. Bend your knee again while returning to the starting position.

PRECAUTION

Carry out the leg press with a smooth and controlled motion, avoiding sudden or forceful movements. If you experience discomfort, adjust the resistance band tension or range of motion accordingly.

SEATED HIP HIKES

Seated Hip Hikes are a targeted exercise designed to engage the muscles in the hips and thighs while promoting stability and strength in the lower body. This seated movement is particularly beneficial for individuals seeking to enhance their hip flexor strength and improve overall mobility.

Repetitions: 20 times per side

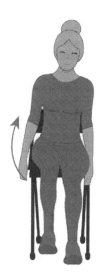 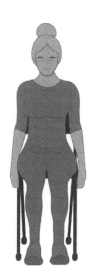 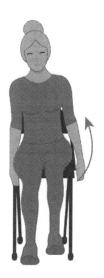

MUSCLES TARGETED

- Hip abductors (outer thigh muscles)
- Hip flexors
- Quadriceps

INSTRUCTIONS

1. Sit in your chair comfortably with an upright posture and make sure that your back is straight and shoulders are relaxed.

2. Place your feet flat on the floor, hip-width apart.

3. Engage your core muscles to stabilize your torso.

4. Lift your right hip by lifting your right foot a few inches off the ground while keeping your knee bent.

5. Lower your right foot back to the floor and repeat the motion on the left side, lift your left hip.

6. Continue this alternating hip hiking motion, creating a controlled lift and lower of each hip.

7. Try to match the pace of your movement with the breath while inhaling as you lift and exhaling as you lower.

8. Keep your pace smooth and deliberate during the exercise.

PRECAUTION

Carry out the seated hip hikes with controlled movements, avoiding any sudden or forceful actions.

SEATED KNEE CIRCLES WITH EXTENSION

Seated Knee Circles with Extension is a versatile exercise that combines knee circles with leg extensions, promoting flexibility and strength in the lower body. This seated routine is suitable for individuals looking to improve hip mobility, engage the quadriceps and enhance overall leg function.

Repetitions: 15 times in each direction

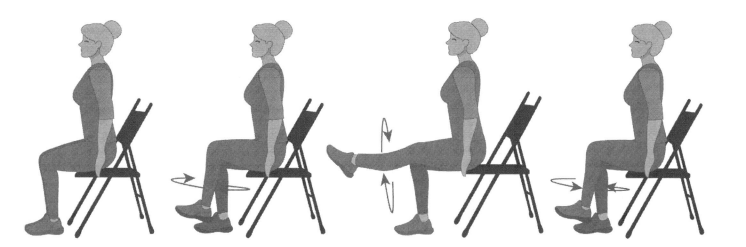

MUSCLES TARGETED

- Hip flexors
- Quadriceps
- Hamstrings

INSTRUCTIONS

1. Sit in your chair, in a comfortable position, with your back straight and shoulders relaxed.

2. Place your feet flat on the floor, hip-width apart.

3. Lift your right knee towards your chest, creating a circular motion with your knee.

4. Extend your right leg straight out in front of you, engaging your quadriceps.

5. Return your right foot to the floor and continue the circular motion in the opposite direction.

6. Repeat the knee circles with the extension on the left leg.

7. Continue to switch between knee circles and leg extensions, creating a fluid and controlled movement.

8. Try to match the pace of your movement with the breath.

PRECAUTION

Practice the seated knee circles with extension with controlled movements, avoiding any sudden or forceful actions to prevent strain on the knee joints.

SEATED QUADRATUS LUMBORUM STRETCH

Seated Quadratus Lumborum Stretch is a targeted exercise designed to alleviate tension in the lower back and promote flexibility in the quadratus lumborum muscle. This seated stretch is especially beneficial for individuals looking to address discomfort or stiffness in the lower back area.

Repetitions: Hold each stretch for 50 seconds per side

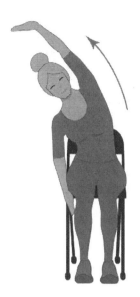 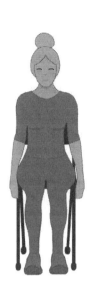 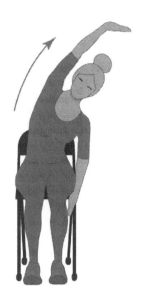

MUSCLES TARGETED

- Quadratus lumborum
- Low back muscles

INSTRUCTIONS

1. Sit in your chair, in a comfortable position, with your back straight and shoulders relaxed.

2. Place your feet flat on the floor, hip-width apart.

3. Engage your core muscles to maintain an upright posture.

4. While seated, lean slightly to your right and bring your right hand to the outside of your right hip.

5. Extend your left arm overhead and reach towards the right side, creating a gentle stretch along the left side of your torso.

6. Hold the stretch for 50 seconds, feeling a comfortable pull along the left side.

7. Return to an upright position and repeat the stretch on the opposite side, leaning to the left while reaching your right arm overhead.

PRECAUTION

Carry out the Quadratus Lumborum Stretch with gradual and controlled movements, avoiding any sudden or forceful actions.

SEATED LEG CROSS HIP LIFTS

Seated Leg Cross Hip Lifts provide a focused workout for seniors, targeting the hip flexors and core muscles while seated. This exercise helps improve lower body strength and stability.

Repetitions: 8 times per leg

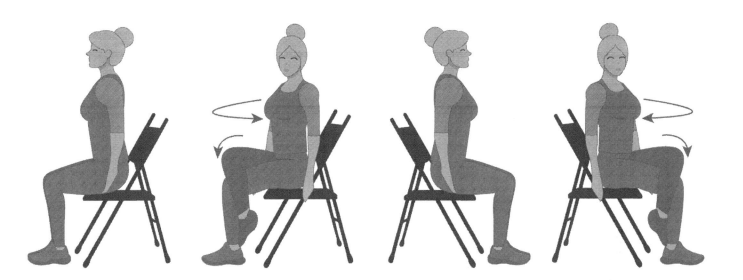

MUSCLES TARGETED

- Hip flexors
- Abductor muscles
- Core muscles

INSTRUCTIONS

1. Comfortably, sit in your chair with your back straight and shoulders relaxed.

2. Keep your feet flat on the floor, maintaining hip-width apart.

3. Lift your right leg and cross it over your left leg, creating a slight twist in your torso.

4. Lower your right leg back to the starting position.

5. Lift your left leg and cross it over your right leg, engaging your core.

6. Repeat the leg cross-motion, alternating between the right and left legs.

7. Coordinate the movement with your breath, exhaling as you lift and inhaling as you lower.

8. Keep your pace controlled and focus on the contraction of the hip and core muscles.

PRECAUTION

Execute Seated Leg Cross Hip Lifts with care and keep smooth and controlled movements to prevent any strain.

SEATED DYNAMIC ARM CIRCLES WITH HIP MOVEMENT

Seated Dynamic Arm Circles with Hip Movement is a rejuvenating exercise designed to enhance upper body flexibility and engage the hip muscles. This seated routine incorporates dynamic arm circles alongside coordinated hip movements, making it a well-rounded exercise suitable for individuals looking to improve overall mobility.

Repetitions: 8 times (4 circles in each direction)

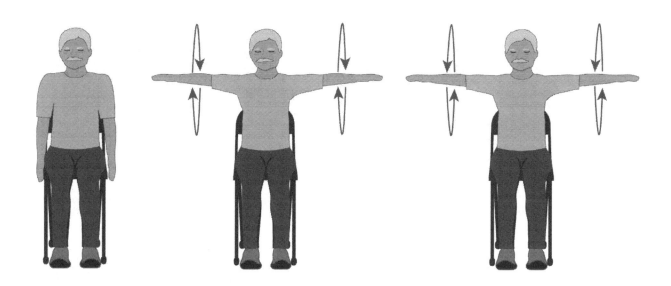

MUSCLES TARGETED

- Shoulders
- Triceps
- Upper back
- Hip abductors and adductors

INSTRUCTIONS

1. Sit in your chair comfortably with an upright posture and relaxed shoulders.

2. Place your feet flat on the floor, hip-width apart.

3. Extend your arms straight out to the sides at shoulder height.

4. Initiate a circular motion with your arms, making controlled circles in a clockwise direction.

5. Coordinate the arm circles with gentle movements of your hips, swaying them side to side.

6. After completing the clockwise circles, reverse the direction and perform anticlockwise circles.

7. Continue the coordinated arm and hip movements for the designated repetitions.

PRECAUTION

Carry out the arm circles and hip movements in a controlled manner and avoid any sudden or jerky motions to prevent strain or injury.

28-DAY ADVANCED CHAIR YOGA CHALLENGE

WEEK 01

Days	Warm-Up	Heart Health	Bad posture	Weight-loss	Joint Mobility
Monday	kundalini circles (seated torso circles) **p.76**	Seated Star Pose **p.79**	Seated Ribcage Side Stretch **p.84**	Seated Torso Twist Punches **p.89**	Leg Press **p.68**
Tuesday	Half Lift (Ardha Uttanasana) **p.74**	Seated Eagle Arms **p.80**	Chest Press **p.85**	Seated Leg Cross and Reach **p.90**	Seated Hip Hikes **p.96**
Wednesday	Cobra Pose (Bhujangasana) **p.75**	Seated Warrior III **p.81**	Seated Lateral Band **p.86**	Seated Mountain Pose with Arm Reach **p.91**	Seated Knee Circles with Extension **p.97**
Thursday	Seated Shoulder Stretch **p.77**	Seated Figure Four Stretch **p.82**	Seated Chin Tucks **p.87**	Seated Knee Lifts with Twist **p.92**	Seated Quadratus Lumborum Stretch **p.98**
Friday	Seated Heel Slides **p.78**	Seated Mountain Climbers **p.83**	Seated Rhomboid Squeeze **p.88**	Seated Quadriceps Activation **p.93**	Seated Leg Cross Hip Lifts **p.99**
Saturday	Half Lift (Ardha Uttanasana) **p.74**	Seated Star Pose **p.79**	Seated Ribcage Side Stretch **p.84**	Seated Lateral Arm Raises with Leg Cross **p.94**	Seated Dynamic Arm Circles with Hip Movement **p.100**
Sunday	Cobra Pose (Bhujangasana) **p.75**	Seated Eagle Arms **p.80**	Chest Press **p.85**	Seated Torso Twist Punches **p.89**	Leg Press **p.68**

WEEK 02

Days	Warm-Up	Heart Health	Bad posture	Weight-loss	Joint Mobility
Monday	Half Lift (Ardha Uttanasana) **p.74**	Seated Warrior III **p.81**	Seated Lateral Band **p.86**	Seated Mountain Pose with Arm Reach **p.91**	Seated Quadratus Lumborum Stretch **p.98**
Tuesday	Cobra Pose (Bhujangasana) **p.75**	Seated Mountain Climbers **p.83**	Seated Chin Tucks **p.87**	Seated Knee Lifts with Twist **p.92**	Seated Leg Cross Hip Lifts **p.99**
Wednesday	Seated Shoulder Stretch **p.77**	Seated Star Pose **p.79**	Seated Rhomboid Squeeze **p.88**	Seated Quadriceps Activation **p.93**	Seated Dynamic Arm Circles with Hip Movement **p.100**
Thursday	Seated Heel Slides **p.78**	Seated Eagle Arms **p.80**	Seated Ribcage Side Stretch **p.84**	Seated Lateral Arm Raises with Leg Cross **p.94**	Seated Quadratus Lumborum Stretch **p.98**
Friday	Half Lift (Ardha Uttanasana) **p.74**	Seated Warrior III **p.81**	Chest Press **p.85**	Seated Torso Twist Punches **p.89**	Leg Press **p.68**
Saturday	Cobra Pose (Bhujangasana) **p.75**	Seated Figure Four Stretch **p.82**	Seated Lateral Band **p.86**	Seated Leg Cross and Reach **p.90**	Seated Hip Hikes **p.96**
Sunday	kundalini circles (seated torso circles) **p.76**	Seated Mountain Climbers **p.83**	Seated Chin Tucks **p.87**	Seated Mountain Pose with Arm Reach **p.91**	Seated Knee Circles with Extension **p.97**

The Only Chair Yoga for Seniors Over 60 Guide You Need

WEEK 03

Days	Warm-Up	Heart Health	Bad posture	Weight-loss	Joint Mobility
Monday	Seated Shoulder Stretch **p.77**	Seated Star Pose **p.79**	Seated Ribcage Side Stretch **p.84**	Seated Torso Twist Punches **p.89**	Leg Press **p.68**
Tuesday	kundalini circles (seated torso circles) **p.76**	Seated Eagle Arms **p.80**	Chest Press **p.85**	Seated Leg Cross and Reach **p.90**	Seated Hip Hikes **p.96**
Wednesday	Half Lift (Ardha Uttanasana) **p.74**	Seated Warrior III **p.81**	Seated Lateral Band **p.86**	Seated Mountain Pose with Arm Reach **p.91**	Seated Knee Circles with Extension **p.97**
Thursday	Cobra Pose (Bhujangasana) **p.75**	Seated Figure Four Stretch **p.82**	Seated Chin Tucks **p.87**	Seated Knee Lifts with Twist **p.92**	Seated Quadratus Lumborum Stretch **p.98**
Friday	Seated Shoulder Stretch **p.77**	Seated Mountain Climbers **p.83**	Seated Rhomboid Squeeze **p.88**	Seated Quadriceps Activation **p.93**	Seated Leg Cross Hip Lifts **p.99**
Saturday	Seated Heel Slides **p.78**	Seated Star Pose **p.79**	Seated Ribcage Side Stretch **p.84**	Seated Lateral Arm Raises with Leg Cross **p.94**	Seated Dynamic Arm Circles with Hip Movement **p.100**
Sunday	Half Lift (Ardha Uttanasana) **p.74**	Seated Eagle Arms **p.80**	Chest Press **p.85**	Seated Torso Twist Punches **p.89**	Leg Press **p.68**

WEEK 04

Days	Warm-Up	Heart Health	Bad posture	Weight-loss	Joint Mobility
Monday	Half Lift (Ardha Uttanasana) **p.74**	Seated Mountain Climbers **p.83**	Seated Lateral Band **p.86**	Seated Mountain Pose with Arm Reach **p.91**	Seated Quadratus Lumborum Stretch **p.98**
Tuesday	Cobra Pose (Bhujangasana) **p.75**	Seated Star Pose **p.79**	Seated Chin Tucks **p.87**	Seated Knee Lifts with Twist **p.92**	Seated Leg Cross Hip Lifts **p.99**
Wednesday	Seated Shoulder Stretch **p.77**	Seated Eagle Arms **p.80**	Seated Rhomboid Squeeze **p.88**	Seated Quadriceps Activation **p.93**	Seated Dynamic Arm Circles with Hip Movement **p.100**
Thursday	Seated Heel Slides **p.78**	Seated Warrior III **p.81**	Seated Lateral Band **p.86**	Seated Lateral Arm Raises with Leg Cross **p.94**	Seated Quadratus Lumborum Stretch **p.98**
Friday	Half Lift (Ardha Uttanasana) **p.74**	Seated Figure Four Stretch **p.82**	Seated Chin Tucks **p.87**	Seated Torso Twist Punches **p.89**	Leg Press **p.68**
Saturday	kundalini circles (seated torso circles) **p.76**	Seated Mountain Climbers **p.83**	Seated Ribcage Side Stretch **p.84**	Seated Leg Cross and Reach **p.90**	Seated Hip Hikes **p.96**
Sunday	Seated Shoulder Stretch **p.77**	Seated Star Pose **p.79**	Chest Press **p.85**	Seated Mountain Pose with Arm Reach **p.91**	Seated Knee Circles with Extension **p.97**

The Only Chair Yoga for Seniors Over 60 Guide You Need

CHAPTER 6:
MIND-BODY CONNECTION THROUGH CHAIR YOGA

"Aging is not lost youth but a new stage of opportunity and strength."
- Betty Friedan

We are as strong as our neural connections. The better the mind-body connection we have the stronger we feel. While chair yoga has a direct physical impact, it is equally beneficial to cultivate a healthy relationship between the mind and body by combining gentle physical movements with mindful breathing and mental focus. Through conscious awareness of body sensations, breath and thoughts, you can deepen your understanding of your inner self and develop a sense of unity between mind, body and spirit. This integrated and holistic approach not only enhances physical health but also alleviates stress, anxiety and depression.

MEDITATION TECHNIQUES FOR SENIORS

What is Meditation? It is a time-tested practice that trains the mind to focus and redirect thoughts which leads you to a heightened state of awareness and inner peace. It is a century-old practice and it can be traced back to thousands of years to ancient Eastern traditions, like Hinduism and Buddhism, where it was used as a tool for spiritual growth and self-discovery. In meditation, you sit quietly in a comfortable position, close your eyes and focus your attention on a specific object, thought or sensation, such as the breath or a mantra. Through regular practice, meditation can leave profound effects on the mind-body connection. It can reduce stress and anxiety levels, improve concentration and memory, enhance emotional regulation and promote overall well-being. Meditation can be practiced in different ways:

Seated Meditation: You can practice meditation comfortably seated in your chair with good back support or on a cushion. Sit upright and focus on your breath or an object of meditation such as the visual of a flowing water body.

Guided Meditation: In guided meditation, you don't rely on your imagination, instead you listen to a voice with your eyes closed and then you follow the verbal instruction and guidance to a visual and think accordingly. You can find numerous guided meditation recordings available online or through apps that cater to individual's needs and preferences.

Mindful Walking: In walking meditation, you pay attention to each step and the sensations of walking. You can practice this in a safe and comfortable environment, such as a garden or a quiet indoor space while focusing on the movement of your feet and the rhythm of your breath.

Breathing Exercises: Seniors can engage in simple breathing exercises to promote relaxation and reduce stress. Techniques such as deep belly breathing or alternate nostril breathing can help calm the mind and body.

Body Scan Meditation: This technique is used to systematically bring awareness to different parts of the body, noticing any sensations without judgment. You can do a seated or lying down body scan, starting from your toes and gradually moving up to your head.

Loving-Kindness Meditation (Metta): Metta meditation is all about cultivating feelings of love, compassion and kindness towards oneself and others. You can repeat phrases such as "May I be happy, may I be healthy, may I be safe," extending these wishes to loved ones, caregivers and all beings.

Nature Meditation: You can connect with nature through this meditation by sitting outside or near a window and observing the sights, sounds and sensations of the natural world. This can help develop a sense of peace and interconnectedness.

Gratitude Meditation: Practicing gratitude is another form of meditation that can enhance your well-being and sense of contentment. You can take a few moments each day to reflect on things you are grateful for, whether it is simple pleasures, cherished memories or the support of loved ones.

Visualization Meditation: You can engage in visualization techniques to imagine yourself in peaceful and serene settings, such as a beach or a tranquil garden. You can visualize details like the sights, sounds and smells and allow yourself to relax deeply into the visualization.

DAILY CHAIR YOGA AND MEDITATION INTEGRATION

A healthy and productive routine has a mix of chair yoga and meditation exercises. Together these exercises create a powerful duo that works like magic in improving physical and mental well-being. Here is just a basic template to give an idea of how you can incorporate chair yoga and meditation into your daily routine. You can customize it as per your schedule and daily needs:

Morning:

First, wake up and start your day with 5-minute stretch. Begin the day with gentle stretching while seated in a chair. Exercises like arms reach overhead, side bends and neck and shoulder rolls are perfect in this regard to release any stiffness from muscles after sleep.

Once you are done with stretches or the warm-up exercise, you can switch to breathing exercises to relax your body and mind. Practice deep breathing exercises to energize the body and calm the mind. Select any of the breathing exercises from this chapter and practice them for 2-3 minutes.

After the relaxation, go for a full-on chair yoga session which may extend up to 15-20 minutes. Start a chair yoga session focusing on gentle movements and stretches. Add poses such as seated jumping jacks, forward folds and gentle twists to promote flexibility and circulation.

Midday:

This is the time of the day when you need to introduce mindful eating for 5-10 minutes. While having your lunch, savor each bite, pay attention to the flavors, textures and sensations of the food to sharpen your senses and focus.

Take a break from and go out for a walk for 15 minutes. Walk slowly and mindfully and pay attention to each step and the sensations in your body.

Afternoon:

In the afternoon you can then take a yoga break for 5-10 minutes. At this point, start a brief chair yoga session to get relief from sitting for extended periods. Focus on gentle stretches for the neck, shoulders and hips to alleviate tension and improve posture.

Then begin a gratitude meditation session to reflect on things you are thankful for. Encourage yourself to cultivate feelings of appreciation and contentment and develop a positive outlook on life.

Evening:

Lastly, in the evening go for relaxation Meditation of 10-15 minutes. A guided relaxation meditation can help you unwind and prepare for sleep. With a body scan or progressive muscle relaxation, let yourself release tension and find deep relaxation.

Lastly, end your day with a bedtime yoga routine for 5 minutes. This yoga routine has to be short and calming to promote relaxation and ease any remaining tension in the body. Practice gentle stretches and restorative poses that can be done while lying in bed or seated on the edge of the bed.

BREATHING PRACTICE
WHICH IMPACTS BETTER SLEEPING

Breathing practices hold paramount importance as they serve as a basic tool for regulating the body's physiological responses and developing a deeper connection between the mind and body. Conscious breathing techniques, such as deep diaphragmatic breathing or mindful breathing, can induce a state of relaxation, reduce stress levels and promote overall mental well-being. By directing attention to the breath, you can anchor yourself in the present moment, alleviate anxiety and promote clarity of thought. Some common breathing exercises that you can add to your yoga routine include:

Deep Belly Breathing (Diaphragmatic Breathing): For this, sit or lie down comfortably. Place one hand on your chest and the other on your abdomen. Deeply inhale through your nostrils and allow your abdomen to rise as you fill your lungs with air. Exhale slowly through your mouth and feeling your abdomen fall. Repeat for several breaths.

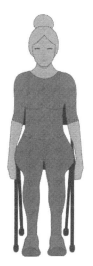 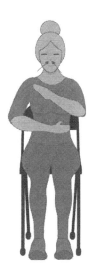 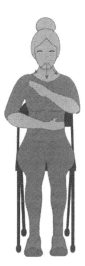

Equal Breathing (Sama Vritti): For this exercise, inhale for a count of four, then exhale for a count of four, maintaining equal lengths for both the inhale and exhale. This breathing exercise promotes balance and calmness.

4-7-8 Breathing: In this exercise you inhale through your nose for a count of four, hold your breath for a count of seven, then exhale slowly through your mouth for a count of eight. This technique is helpful for reducing anxiety and promoting relaxation.

Alternate Nostril Breathing (Nadi Shodhana): Start by sitting comfortably with your spine straight. Use your right thumb to close your right nostril and inhale through your left nostril. Close your left nostril with your right ring finger, release your thumb and exhale through your right nostril. Inhale through your right nostril, close it with your thumb, release your ring finger and exhale through your left nostril. Continue this pattern for several breaths, alternating nostrils.

Box Breathing (Square Breathing): In this technique, you inhale deeply for a count of four, hold your breath for a count of four, exhale completely for a count of four and then hold your breath again for a count of four before beginning the next cycle. Repeat for several rounds.

Rhythmic Breathing: Create a natural rhythm of breathing that feels comfortable for you. Focus on maintaining a steady and consistent pace and allow your breath to flow smoothly without pauses or disruptions.

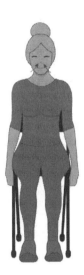 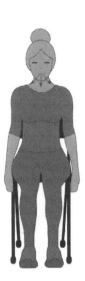

Cleansing Breath (Kapalabhati): Sit comfortably with a straight spine. Take a deep breath in through your nose, then forcefully exhale through your nose while contracting your abdominal muscles. Let the inhalation occur passively. Repeat this rapid exhalation-inhalation cycle for 30 seconds to a minute, then return to normal breathing.

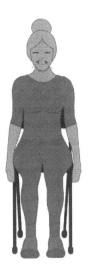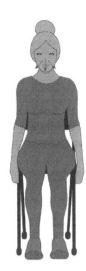

Humming Bee Breath (Bhramari Pranayama): Close your eyes and take a deep breath in. As you exhale, make a humming sound like a bee and allow the sound to be smooth and steady. Feel the vibrations in your head and chest. Repeat for several breaths.

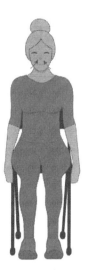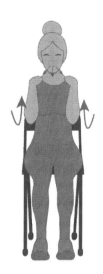

Progressive Muscle Relaxation Breathing: This exercise combines deep breathing with progressive muscle relaxation. Inhale deeply, tensing specific muscle groups (e.g., fists, shoulders) as you breathe in, then exhale and release the tension as you breathe out. Move through different muscle groups, progressively to relax the entire body.

Visualization Breathing: Close your eyes and imagine a peaceful scene or a place where you feel calm and relaxed. As you inhale, visualize yourself breathing in positive energy or light. As you exhale, imagine releasing any tension or negativity. Repeat for several breaths, focusing on the imagery and sensations.

BONUS # 01:
CHAIR YOGA AND HEALTHY NUTRITION

Chair yoga and healthy nutrition go hand-in-hand as they form a harmonious duo for promoting overall well-being. While chair yoga offers a gentle yet effective way to improve flexibility, strength and mental clarity, healthy nutrition provides the essential nutrients needed to support these efforts. A balanced diet rich in fruits, vegetables, lean proteins and whole grains fuels the body with the energy and nutrients necessary for optimal performance during chair yoga sessions. By incorporating both chair yoga and healthy nutrition into their daily routines, you can enhance your physical and mental health, for a more vibrant and fulfilling lifestyle. Together, these practices create a synergistic relationship, promoting holistic wellness from the inside out.

THE ROLE OF NUTRITION IN SENIOR WELL-BEING

As we age, we become more susceptible to deficiencies in essential nutrients and more vulnerable to various diseases. Consuming a healthy diet rich in nutrients becomes crucial during this stage of life to support overall health and well-being. Changes in metabolism, absorption and digestion are quite common at this age and that can lead to nutrient deficiencies if dietary intake is inadequate. For instance, calcium and vitamin D are essential for maintaining bone health and preventing osteoporosis. Adequate intake of vitamins C and E along with zinc and selenium, can help support immune function and reduce the risk of infections. Omega-3 fatty acids found in fish and nuts play a role in brain health and may help prevent cognitive decline associated with aging. A balanced diet that is rich in fruits, vegetables, whole grains, lean proteins and healthy fats is necessary to support the immune system, bone health, cognitive function and overall vitality, Hence, it reduces the risk of age-related diseases.

NUTRITIONAL TIPS

If you want to keep your energy levels high without relying on unhealthy, processed and sugar-rich food products then start consuming healthy snacks in between the meals. Such snacks satisfy your unwanted food cravings, and offer you loads of nutrients and fiber without raising your blood sugar levels. Some good options that you can easily prepare without much effort include:

Fresh Fruit: You can enjoy a variety of fresh fruits such as apples, oranges, bananas, berries or sliced melon as snacks. These ingredients are rich in vitamins, minerals and antioxidants and provide natural sweetness without increasing your calorie count.

Vegetable Sticks with Hummus: Another way to prepare a high-fiber snack is to serve carrot sticks, cucumber slices, bell pepper strips or cherry tomatoes with hummus for a satisfying snack loaded with fiber, vitamins and protein.

Greek Yogurt with Berries: Serve low-fat or Greek yogurt with fresh berries like strawberries, blueberries or raspberries on top. This snack is high in protein, calcium and antioxidants.

Mixed Nuts: You can consume a handful of mixed nuts such as almonds, walnuts or pistachios as a crunchy snack rich in healthy fats, protein and fiber. Since nuts are nutrient-dense they are loaded with calories, so be mindful of the portion sizes while consuming them.

Whole Grain Crackers with Cheese: Add whole grain crackers with sliced cheese to your snack menu. It has a mix of protein, calcium and complex carbohydrates for sustained energy.

Oatmeal with Nut Butter: Oatmeal topped with a dollop of almond butter or peanut butter is another healthy snack option to go for. This snack is nutritious and a good source of fiber and healthy fats.

Cottage Cheese with Pineapple: Cottage cheese with pineapple chunks is another refreshing and protein-rich snack that can provide vitamins and minerals.

Hard-Boiled Eggs: For a protein-rich snack keep a batch of hard-boiled eggs in the fridge and enjoy when you feel like munching. Sprinkle some black pepper and salt on top before consuming for good taste.

Homemade Trail Mix: Trail mixes are made of a combination of unsalted nuts, seeds, dried fruits and whole grain cereal and you can create your own mixture for a nutrient-dense snack.

Smoothies: Smoothies are a complete meal in themselves, you can consume them in the morning or during snack time. Blend a combination of your favorite fruits, leafy greens, yogurt or milk and a scoop of protein powder for a refreshing and nutritious snack that is easy to consume and digest.

HYDRATION

Water plays a central role in regulating body temperature, aiding digestion, transporting nutrients and removing waste products from the body. It helps lubricate joints, cushion organs and support healthy skin. Whereas dehydration can lead to fatigue, headaches, impaired physical performance and even more serious health issues if left untreated. Therefore, it is important to drink water regularly throughout the day, especially during and after physical activity, in hot weather or when experiencing illness. Aim to drink at least 8 glasses of water per day and adjust your intake based on individual factors such as age, weight, activity level and climate.

FOOD TO LIMIT & AVOID:

There are food items that are never good for the physical and mental health of a person, but once you cross the age of 50 keeping those ingredients in your diet becomes more hazardous than ever. So, if you consume any of the following food through your diet then put that on pause right now and start opting better and healthier options.

Processed and Junk Foods: Foods high in processed sugars, unhealthy fats and refined grains should be limited. These foods offer little nutritional value and can contribute to weight gain, inflammation and chronic health conditions such as diabetes and heart disease.

High-Sodium Foods: You need to watch your sodium intake, as excessive salt can lead to high blood pressure, fluid retention and increased risk of stroke and heart disease. Processed foods, canned soups, deli meats and salty snacks are common sources of hidden sodium.

Sugary Snacks and Beverages: You should also minimize the consumption of sugary snacks, desserts and sweetened beverages like soda and fruit juices. These foods can contribute to weight gain, tooth decay and may even exacerbate conditions such as diabetes and inflammation.

Fatty and Fried Foods: Foods high in unhealthy fats, such as saturated and trans fats, should be limited. These fats can raise cholesterol levels and increase the risk of heart disease. Fried foods, fatty meats, full-fat dairy products and processed snacks are examples of foods to avoid or consume in moderation.

Alcohol: While moderate alcohol consumption may be acceptable for some older adults, excessive alcohol intake can pose risks, including liver damage, impaired cognitive function and increased risk of falls and accidents. You should limit alcohol intake and consult with your healthcare provider regarding safe levels of consumption.

NUTRITION FOR ENDURANCE: BALANCED MEALS

A good way to keep all the unhealthy ingredients at bay and meet all your nutritional requirements is to plan your meals and carry out a thoughtful selection of wholesome foods from diverse food groups. Here is how you can curate well-rounded meal for yourself:

Start with whole grains: Kick off the meal with hearty whole grains like brown rice, quinoa or whole wheat pasta, delivering complex carbs, fiber and vital nutrients.

Lean into lean proteins: Lean proteins such as skinless poultry, fish, beans or tofu take center stage as they provide essential muscle-building nutrients while keeping it light on the fats.

Pile on the produce: Load up half the plate with a vibrant range of fruits and veggies. Their colorful palette brings in crucial vitamins, minerals, fiber and antioxidants, promoting immune strength, heart health and smooth digestion.

Add a dash of healthy fats: Sprinkle in sources of healthy fats like nuts, seeds, avocados or olive oil for a flavorful punch that supports brain health, reduces inflammation and keeps the heart happy.

Dabble in dairy: Go for low-fat or fat-free dairy options like milk, yogurt or cheese for a calcium and vitamin D boost and keep those bones strong and sturdy.

Cater to your special needs: Be mindful of any dietary restrictions or special preferences and the meal plan accordingly to accommodate your health requirements. For instance, if you have diabetes then remove all forms of high glycemic (high sugar) food from the diet.

NUTRITION FOR JOINT HEALTH

Nutrition plays a significant role in joint health, particularly in managing inflammation, which is a common factor in conditions such as osteoarthritis and rheumatoid arthritis. Here are some foods that may help decrease inflammation in the joints:

Fatty Fish: Fatty fish like salmon, mackerel, sardines and trout are rich in omega-3 fatty acids, which have anti-inflammatory properties. Consuming fatty fish regularly can help reduce inflammation and alleviate joint pain.

Flaxseeds and Chia Seeds: These seeds are excellent plant-based sources of omega-3 fatty acids. Sprinkling ground flaxseeds or chia seeds on salads, yogurt or oatmeal can provide anti-inflammatory benefits for joint health.

Nuts: Nuts such as almonds, walnuts and pistachios contain healthy fats and antioxidants that help combat inflammation. They can be enjoyed as a snack or added to salads, stir-fries or baked goods.

The Only Chair Yoga for Seniors Over 60 Guide You Need

Berries: Berries like strawberries, blueberries, raspberries and blackberries are rich in antioxidants, particularly flavonoids, which have anti-inflammatory effects. Add a variety of berries to your diet in different ways.

Leafy Green Vegetables: Leafy greens such as spinach, kale, collard greens and Swiss chard are packed with vitamins, minerals and phytonutrients that have anti-inflammatory properties. Incorporate these vegetables into salads, smoothies, soups or stir-fries to promote joint health.

Turmeric: Turmeric contains curcumin, a compound with powerful anti-inflammatory and antioxidant properties. Add turmeric to curries, soups, stews or golden milk to help reduce inflammation and alleviate joint pain.

Ginger: Ginger has been used for centuries for its anti-inflammatory properties. Consuming ginger tea, adding fresh ginger to stir-fries or smoothies or using ground ginger in cooking can help reduce inflammation in the joints.

Extra Virgin Olive Oil: Extra virgin olive oil is rich in monounsaturated fats and antioxidants, including oleocanthal, which has anti-inflammatory effects similar to ibuprofen. Use olive oil as a primary fat source in cooking and salad dressings to support joint health.

Green Tea: Green tea contains catechins, which are antioxidants that have anti-inflammatory effects. Drink green tea regularly to counter inflammation and promote overall health.

Tart Cherry Juice: Tart cherries are rich in anthocyanins, which have potent anti-inflammatory properties. You can drink tart cherry juice or consume whole tart cherries regularly to help decrease inflammation and alleviate joint pain.

TRACKING CHART

28-Days Beginners Challenge

Mark each circle after completing the exercises for the respective day. You can increase the number of repetitions per exercise to meet the suggested time limit for each day in the tracking table.

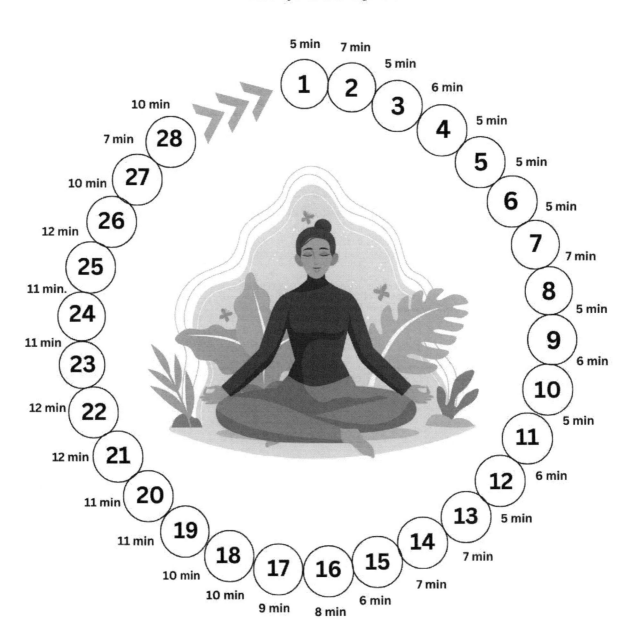

5 min — 1
7 min — 2
5 min — 3
6 min — 4
5 min — 5
5 min — 6
5 min — 7
7 min — 8
5 min — 9
6 min — 10
5 min — 11
6 min — 12
5 min — 13
7 min — 14
7 min — 15
6 min — 16
8 min — 17
9 min — 18
10 min — 19
11 min — 20
12 min — 21
12 min — 22
11 min — 23
11 min. — 24
12 min — 25
10 min — 26
7 min — 27
10 min — 28

28-Day Intermediate Challenge

Mark each circle after completing the exercises for the respective day. You can increase the number of repetitions per exercise to meet the suggested time limit for each day in the tracking table.

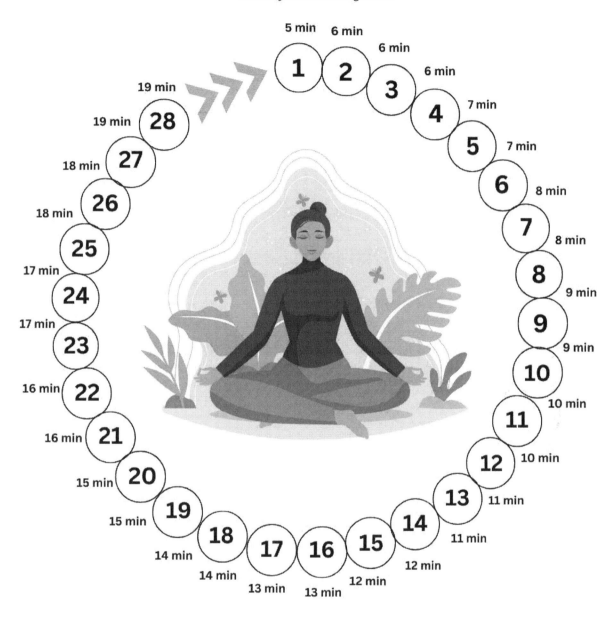

5 min **1**
6 min **2**
6 min **3**
6 min **4**
7 min **5**
7 min **6**
8 min **7**
8 min **8**
9 min **9**
9 min **10**
10 min **11**
10 min **12**
11 min **13**
11 min **14**
12 min **15**
12 min **16**
13 min **17**
13 min **18**
14 min **19**
14 min **20**
15 min **21**
15 min **22**
16 min **23**
16 min **24**
17 min **25**
17 min **26**
18 min **27**
18 min **28**
19 min
19 min

28-Day Advanced Challenge

Mark each circle after completing the exercises for the respective day. You can increase the number of repetitions per exercise to meet the suggested time limit for each day in the tracking table.

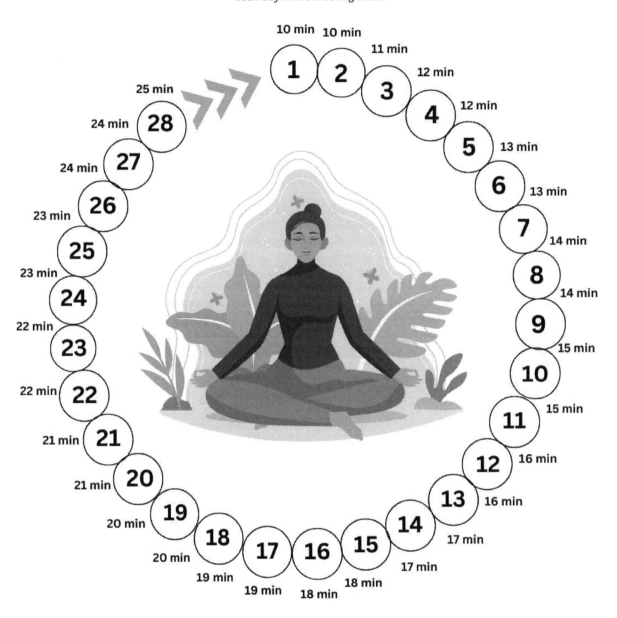

10 min — 1
10 min — 2
11 min — 3
12 min — 4
12 min — 5
13 min — 6
13 min — 7
14 min — 8
14 min — 9
15 min — 10
15 min — 11
16 min — 12
16 min — 13
17 min — 14
17 min — 15
18 min — 16
18 min — 17
19 min — 18
19 min — 19
20 min — 20
20 min — 21
21 min — 22
21 min — 23
22 min — 24
22 min — 25
23 min — 26
23 min — 27
24 min — 28
24 min
25 min

The Only Chair Yoga for Seniors Over 60 Guide You Need

CONCLUSION

Let's take a moment here to celebrate the progress and achievements you made so far on your chair yoga journey. Through the text of this book, we have together explored a variety of chair yoga poses, stretches and exercises that not only increase flexibility but also improve strength with a greater sense of peace and well-being. Every step you take toward healthier living is definitely worth acknowledging and honoring. So, give yourself a pat on the back and pledge to stick to your chair yoga routine to continue your active lifestyle. While you acknowledge your accomplishment, let's look ahead with optimism and determination. The chair yoga practice has the power to enrich your lives in profound ways. So, let's commit to sparing a few minutes every day for practicing breathing exercises, yoga poses and stretches shared in this book and see yourself transforming into a healthier being. With great dedication and perseverance, you can unlock even greater levels of physical, mental and spiritual growth.

YOUR FREE BONUS

As an additional BONUS for your purchase, I would like to give you a GIFT.

This is a BALANCED PLATE for breakfast, lunch and dinner!

BALANCED PLATE- the optimal combination of proteins, fats, carbohydrates, vitamins and trace elements in the diet. It is necessary to ensure the normal functioning of the body, and good well-being at the physical and mental level.

HERE you will get not only nutrition recommendations but also

ready-made recipes for a balanced diet that can be immediately used in your everyday life!

Scan the QR code or follow the link

https://amazon-book.minisite.ai/chairyogabonusforseniors

REFERENCES

Baiera, V. (2021, August 20). *Benefits of Chair Yoga for seniors - Reduce Pain and Improve Health.* Step2Health. https://step2health.com/blogs/news/benefits-of-chair-yoga-for-seniors

Bh, K., & Pal, P. (2014). Effect of yoga therapy on heart rate, blood pressure and cardiac autonomic function in heart failure. *Journal of Clinical and Diagnostic Research.* https://doi.org/10.7860/jcdr/2014/7844.3983

Brenes, G. A., Sohl, S. J., Wells, R. E., Befus, D., Campos, C. L., & Danhauer, S. C. (2019). The Effects of Yoga on Patients with Mild Cognitive Impairment and Dementia: A Scoping Review. *The American Journal of Geriatric Psychiatry*, 27(2), 188–197. https://doi.org/10.1016/j.jagp.2018.10.013

Furtado, G. E., Chupel, M. U., Carvalho, H. M., Souza, N. R., Ferreira, J. P., & Teixeira, A. M. (2016). Effects of a chair-yoga exercises on stress hormone levels, daily life activities, falls and physical fitness in institutionalized older adults. *Complementary Therapies in Clinical Practice*, 24, 123–129. https://doi.org/10.1016/j.ctcp.2016.05.012

Home, K. A. (n.d.). *Eight (8) simple breathing exercises for older adults.* https://www.kendalathome.org/blog/breathe-easy-six-breath-exercises-for-older-adults

Jeter, P. E., Nkodo, A., Moonaz, S., & Dagnelie, G. (2014). A Systematic Review of Yoga for Balance in a Healthy population. *Journal of Alternative and Complementary Medicine*, 20(4), 221–232. https://doi.org/10.1089/acm.2013.0378

Klempel, N., Blackburn, N. E., McMullan, I., Wilson, J. J., Smith, L., Cunningham, C., O'Sullivan, R., Caserotti, P., & Tully, M. A. (2021). The Effect of Chair-Based Exercise on Physical Function in Older Adults: A Systematic Review and Meta-Analysis. *International Journal of Environmental Research and Public Health*, 18(4), 1902. https://doi.org/10.3390/ijerph18041902

Lehmkuhl, L. (2020). *Chair yoga for seniors: Stretches and Poses that You Can Do Sitting Down at Home.* Simon and Schuster.

Lifestyle, S. (2021, October 25). Top 10 chair yoga Positions for Seniors [Infographic]. *Senior Lifestyle.* https://www.seniorlifestyle.com/resources/blog/infographic-top-10-chair-yoga-positions-for-seniors/

Lifestyle, S. (2023, January 3). 10 Healthy benefits of meditation for Seniors - Senior Lifestyle. *Senior Lifestyle.* https://www.seniorlifestyle.com/resources/blog/healthy-benefits-of-meditation-for-seniors/

Park, J., & McCaffrey, R. (2012). Chair Yoga: Benefits for Community-Dwelling Older Adults with Osteoarthritis. *Journal of Gerontological Nursing*, 38(5), 12–22. https://doi.org/10.3928/00989134-20120410-01

Singh, A., Aitken, D., Moonaz, S., Palmer, A. J., Blizzard, L., Ding, C., Drummen, S. J. J., Jones, G., Bennell, K. L., & Antony, B. (2022). A Randomized Controlled Trial of YOGA and Strengthening Exercise for Knee OsteoArthritis: Protocol for a Comparative Effectiveness Trial (YOGA Trial). *Journal of Functional Morphology and Kinesiology*, 7(4), 84. https://doi.org/10.3390/jfmk7040084

Team, M. (2023, August 23). *Best meditation techniques for Seniors.* Mindworks. https://mindworks.org/blog/best-meditation-techniques-seniors/

Yao, C., Lee, B., Hong, H., & Su, Y. (2023). Effect of Chair Yoga Therapy on Functional Fitness and Daily Life Activities among Older Female Adults with Knee Osteoarthritis in Taiwan: A Quasi-Experimental Study. *Healthcare*, 11(7), 1024. https://doi.org/10.3390/healthcare11071024

Yoga for seniors + 5 breathing exercises (Pranayama) for older adults. (2022, August 31). *Prana Sutra Yoga*. https://www.prana-sutra.com/post/yoga-pranayama-for-seniors-older-adults

Made in United States
Troutdale, OR
10/26/2024